WO

T

Ol

Ars

Please return/renew this item by the last date shown

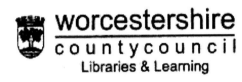
worcestershire
countycouncil
Libraries & Learning

Old-Fashioned Remedies from Arsenic to Gin

Dr Rob Hicks

First published in Great Britain in 2009 by
REMEMBER WHEN
An imprint of
Pen & Sword Books Ltd
47 Church Street
Barnsley
South Yorkshire
S70 2AS

Copyright © Dr Rob Hicks 2009

ISBN 978 1 84468 062 7

The right of Dr Rob Hicks to be identified as Author of this work has been asserted by
him in accordance with the Copyright, Designs and Patents Act 1988.

A CIP catalogue record for this book is available from the British Library

Typeset by Phoenix Typesetting, Auldgirth, Dumfriesshire
Printed and bound by 1010 Printing International

Pen & Sword Books Ltd incorporates the Imprints of Pen & Sword Aviation,
Pen & Sword Maritime, Pen & Sword Military, Wharncliffe Local History,
Pen & Sword Select, Pen & Sword Military Classics,
Leo Cooper, Remember When, Seaforth Publishing and Frontline Publishing.

For a complete list of Pen & Sword titles please contact
PEN & SWORD BOOKS LIMITED
47 Church Street, Barnsley, South Yorkshire, S70 2AS, England
E-mail: enquiries@pen-and-sword.co.uk
Website: www.pen-and-sword.co.uk

Contents

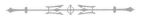

Introduction   1

Section One: Old-Fashioned Remedies
Aloe vera   4
Apple   6
Arnica   9
Bananas   12
Basil   15
Bay leaf   18
Bicarbonate of soda   21
Brown sugar   24
Cabbage   27
Calendula   30
Camomile   33
Carrots   36
Cloves   39
Coconut oil   41
Cranberry   44
Cucumber   47
Epsom salts   50
Feverfew   52
Figs   55
Frozen foods   58
Garlic   61
Horseradish   63
Ice   66
Lavender   69
Lemon balm   72
Lemon juice   75
Liquorice   78
Oatmeal   81
Onions   84
Papaya   87

Peppermint   90
Potato   93
Radish   96
Rolling pin   98
Salt   101
Tea bags   104
Thyme   107
Tomato   110
Tonic water   113
Turmeric   115
Vinegar   118
Witch hazel   121
Yogurt   124
No longer used   127

Section Two: Health Ailments

Acne   130
Alzheimer's disease   131
Anal fissure   131
Anxiety   132
Arthritis   133
Asthma   134
Athlete's foot   135
Back pain   135
Bad breath   136
Blisters   137
Bloating   138
High blood pressure   138
Body odour   139
Breast tenderness   140
Bronchitis   141
Bruises   142
Burns   143
Chapped lips   144
Chickenpox   144
Chilblains   145
Cold sores   146
Constipation   146
Corns and calluses   147
Coughs and colds   148
Cradle cap   150
Croup   150

Cuts and grazes	151
Cystitis	151
Dandruff	152
Depression	153
Diarrhoea	153
Dry skin	154
Eczema	155
Eye bags	156
Fever	157
Foot problems	157
Gout	158
Haemorrhoids	160
Hangover	161
Hayfever	161
Headaches	162
Heart disease	164
Hiccups	164
High cholesterol	165
Impetigo	165
Indigestion	166
Insect bites and stings	167
Insomnia	168
Irritable bowel syndrome	169
Joint problems	169
Laryngitis	171
Leg cramps	172
Poor libido	173
Migraine	173
Morning sickness	175
Mouth ulcers	175
Muscle problems	176
Nasal congestion	178
Nausea and vomiting	179
Neuralgia	179
Nosebleeds	180
Palpitations	181
Period pain	181
Premenstrual syndrome (PMS)	182
Prickly heat	183
Psoriasis	184
Raynaud's phenomenon	185
Razor burn	185

Ringworm	186
Seborrhoeic dermatitis	186
Skin irritation	187
Snoring	188
Sore eyes	189
Sore throat	190
Splinter	191
Stomach ulcer	191
Stress	192
Stretch marks	193
Stroke	194
Stye	194
Sunburn	195
Sweaty feet	196
Thrush	197
Tired eyes	197
Tiredness	198
Toothache	199
Travel sickness	200
Varicose veins	200
Warts and verrucas	201
Waxy ears	202
Wind	203

Index　　　　205

Introduction

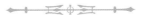

When I was growing up, my family often used natural remedies from our garden or kitchen. This wasn't because they were particularly passionate about these, or against any other kind of medicine. It was because that's what they had grown up with as in those days the belief was you didn't trouble the doctor unless something was serious. So in effect, to use what was available around the home was the norm.

Without being consciously aware of it as a child I was learning about how things around the home could help treat minor ailments. With the passage of time medical school taught me well about disease and conventional treatments, and my patients and others I've had the privilege to meet along the way have taught me about the role of non-drug therapies and

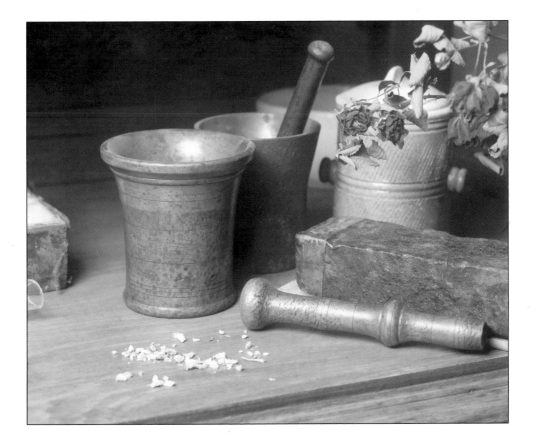

remedies such that I now have what I call my basket of treatments to offer my patients and to make use of at home when needed. This basket has the options of conventional drug treatments, complementary therapies and other natural remedies.

As a doctor with a scientific background, but with a strong belief that treatments other than drugs can help to treat minor ailments, I've often debated with others, and myself for that matter, what is best. I confess it's sometimes been difficult to find anywhere on the fence that's comfortable to sit. On the one hand my scientific brain argues many traditional home-made remedies have no scientific research to support them. On the other hand my experience tells me many of these remedies can help.

Some of the remedies in this book have science behind them, others don't. Some I have used myself, others I have learned about from family, friends, and my patients who have been kind enough to share them with me. My philosophy is this. Even if science hasn't proved a remedy works, provided an individual understands this and that any positive effects may be placebo – as there is with conventional and complementary treatments alike – and importantly, using the remedy isn't going to cause harm, and that an individual isn't being misled, taken advantage of, or ripped off, then there's little harm in giving it a go.

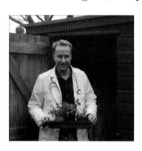

My belief is we should let common sense prevail. After all, they say that medicine is an art, not a science, and for me most of health and medicine is actually more about common sense than anything else. Make use of a dose of common sense and you are unlikely to go far wrong.

I have enjoyed writing this book and I truly hope that you enjoy reading it and find it helpful when, as happens to us all, minor ailments come your way.

CAUTION:
The remedies described in this book should not be used:

- If you have an allergy to any of the ingredients.
- If you already have an existing health problem or are taking medication, without first seeking the advice of your doctor.
- To treat children or babies, unless where specifically described as being safe to do so, without first seeking the advice of your child's or baby's doctor.
- When pregnant or breastfeeding, unless where specifically described as being safe to do so, without first seeking the advice of your doctor.

Before using any of the remedies perform a test dose by applying some of the remedy, in particular those to be applied to the skin, to an area of the skin – inside the upper arm is ideal – to establish whether it is likely to trigger an unwanted reaction.

Always seek medical advice if you have any unexplained symptoms or if a health problem is not getting better or is getting worse despite treatment.

DISCLAIMER:

Old-Fashioned Remedies is intended to inform, entertain, and provoke the thinking of the reader. It is provided for general information only, and should not be treated as a substitute for the medical advice of your own doctor or other health care professional. Whilst every effort has been made to provide accurate and up-to-date information, medical science is constantly evolving. Neither the author nor the publisher can be held responsible or liable for any loss or claim arising out of the use, or misuse, of the suggestions made in this book. We don't know your specific circumstances and so we're not suggesting any specific course of action for you to follow. It's your health, it's your life and so it makes sense for you to weigh up carefully the choices available and to decide what action, if any, you might take. If in doubt you should always consult your doctor for individualised health and medical advice.

Old-Fashioned Remedies

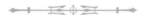

Aloe vera

The 'miracle plant', 'natural healer', or 'first aid plant', aloe vera is known throughout the world by many different names. Cheekily it's also known as the 'cleanser' because of its effect on the bowel. The word 'vera' means 'true' or 'genuine' and that's why I like to think of aloe vera as one of the family, 'Aunt Vera'. Why? Because like an aunt aloe vera soothes and comforts and is wise in so many ways. So, join me in saying, 'hello Vera'.

About aloe vera

Aloe vera with its fleshy and cactus-like long leaves is actually a member of the lily family and is a plant that offers great therapeutic benefits. Slice the leaf open and the gel can be used to help relieve uncomfortable and irritated skin. I wish I'd known this many years ago when by chance I was first introduced to aloe vera.

I was fortunate to be spending some time on the beautiful island of Tobago at the end of my medical elective period – this is officially a chance to study overseas, but in reality it's a chance to have a nice long vacation. I don't feel guilty about coming clean about this because what faced me on my return to the UK were months of days and nights studying for final examinations. Anyway, I digress. On a sun-drenched beach a local vendor approached me carrying armfuls of long, sword-like leaves. He offered me one. To cut a potentially long story short, we had an amicable misunderstanding. Being aware of local culture but never having seen marijuana, and not wishing to get into a bartering situation – I'm British after all and we are no good at bartering are we? – I quickly and without further conversation politely declined his offer. Of course, he had noticed my sunburned skin, and was offering the aloe to me to treat the discomfort that would occur later. We both lost out; him a sale, and me relief from my sunburn.

Scientific research findings regarding aloe vera gel and its health benefits are controversial. Some research demonstrates benefits with, for example skin wound healing, whilst other research contradicts this. One piece of research suggested that when taken internally by those with the inflammatory bowel disease ulcerative colitis it helps lessen the symptoms and the gut cell damage that causes these. Many with irritable bowel syndrome anecdotally report experiencing fewer symptoms when taking the gel internally. Scientific research has confirmed the effects of taking aloe vera juice – extracted from the tubules just beneath the outer skin of the leaves – is an effective laxative, not that anyone who uses it in this way needs research to confirm this.

Did you know?
You can grow aloe vera at home so long as you provide it with suitable conditions. It likes well-drained sandy soil, and grows well in a rockery, or a terracotta pot will do nicely.

Aloe vera history

Aloe vera is widely believed to have originally come from Africa, where the warm and dry climate was perfect for its growth. Its healing benefits are thought to have been documented as long ago as 2200BC and in the Egyptian Papyrus ebers, written around 1550BC, are twelve formulas for mixing aloe with other constituents to treat internal and external disease. Alexander the Great recognised the value of aloe and used it to treat the wounds of his soldiers. But the benefits of aloe vera went further than its medicinal role as Egyptian Queens would use it to beautify themselves.

From this time the external benefit of aloe in relieving skin irritation and its internal benefits as a laxative, described over the years as 'loosening the belly' and 'internal cleansing', became well recognised as they remain to this day.

These days aloe appears in many commercial products including hair-care products, tissues, some foods (yogurts and beverages), and creams where it's used to help improve the quality of hair and skin and treat minor ailments. In fact, I recently found that my wife had brought home toilet tissue infused with aloe. I'm not aware of any scientific research saying that aloe vera impregnated toilet tissue helps but my experience is that it's very soft!

Aloe vera remedies

- **Minor burns** – After running under cold water, apply aloe vera gel to the burn. This can help to speed up healing and lessen the chance of a scar
- **Haemorrhoids** – Apply aloe vera to the affected part after opening the bowels and wiping the area, and apply an additional couple of times during the day

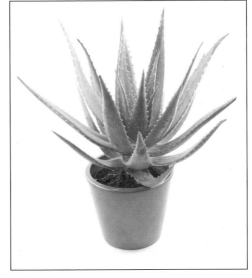

'Allo Vera'

- **Constipation** – Taking the juice of the aloe vera plant helps to relieve constipation by stimulating the bowel to move the stool along, and by possibly softening the stool to make movement easier. It's believed to be chemicals called anthraquinone glycosides in the aloe that are responsible for this action
- **Irritable bowel syndrome** – Some people benefit from taking aloe vera gel to relieve or prevent the symptoms of irritable bowel syndrome
- **Congestion** – Boil one or two aloe vera leaves in water and then inhale the steam to clear blocked nasal passages and sinuses
- **Mouth ulcers and cold sores** – After washing the hands rub fresh aloe vera gel against the mouth ulcer or cold sore. Do this a couple of times a day. Always wash hands afterwards

Fighting sore skin
Aloe vera can hydrate, moisturise and rejuvenate skin when applied to the skin daily. It is thought to stimulate production and regeneration of skin cells responsible for producing collagen, which gives skin its structure, and elastin, which gives skin its elasticity. To relieve the discomfort of itchy, sore, and dry skin apply fresh aloe vera gel to the affected area and gently rub in.

Conclusion

It case you haven't guessed it yet, I'm a great fan of aloe vera. Today, it's available in tubes and other containers, so it's not absolutely necessary to have this vital part of your first-aid kit growing in your garden or as a houseplant, but this has its advantages since it's a very attractive plant to look at.

Even if you do have a plant, do also have a tube of aloe vera in your travel bag because you can't really cart 'Vera' around with you. Although you could carry a leaf the gel is best when fresh and with modern security fears there'll probably be a few concerns about you carrying a sword-like, serrated-edged item at an airport, even if you do say it's for medical purposes, and considered an auntie.

APPLE

'An apple a day keeps the doctor away', and apparently may keep the dentist away too. When it comes to apples and promoting their many health benefits we're halfway there because unlike some less common foods apples are universally known and recognised, often coming top of the pile when people are asked to name their favourite fruit. All in all, the apple is a fruit with tremendous nutritional benefits and many ways to help us out with health problems that arise from time to time.

About Apples

I think it may be fair to say that we take apples for granted. At the supermarket or grocery shop all we have to do is reach into the display and put them into our basket. Sometimes we're able to pick them from heavily laden apple trees, which I did recently with my daughter. What fun we had with the apple catcher.

We should though spend a moment to marvel at how these delicious and nutritious apples came to be. It takes four to five years before an apple tree produces its first fruit, and to produce just one apple is estimated to take the energy of fifty leaves. So I for one enjoy this wonderful member of the rose

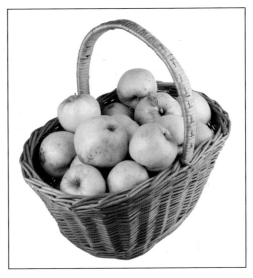

"The doctor's bag"

family, of which there are more than 7,500 different cultivars producing fruits of different shades of green, red, and yellow, in a variety of sizes ranging from as large as a grapefruit to almost as small as a cherry. In fact, some varieties have an aftertaste of other foods, for example, that of pineapple, cinnamon, and even coconut.

Apples contain a soluble fibre called pectin that encourages growth of beneficial bacteria in the gut, the 'friendly bacteria', helping the gut to function well. Pectin may also help to lower cholesterol and glucose levels in the blood which in turn may help protect the heart and circulation from damage. Apples are a good source of vitamin C, fibre, potassium and folic acid, and contain flavonoids and antioxidants that may help improve immune function and prevent heart disease and some cancers.

Although most commonly eaten as the fresh fruit apples are used in many different ways. They are added to salads, baked, used in pies, cakes, and tarts – my Dad has a passion for deep apple pie. They're also covered in sticky toffee, and made into sauces, relishes, juices, and cider. I remember how it came as quite a surprise to find apple in my aunt's lamb casserole. But from that moment this became one of my favourite dishes.

Did you know?

Apples are sodium, fat, and cholesterol-free, and twenty-five per cent of an apple's volume is air – which helps them float when bobbing for apples at Halloween – making them a very healthy and nutritious food. No wonder for years people have repeated the well-known saying, 'an apple a day keeps the doctor away', believed to have originated from 'to eat an apple before going to bed, will make the doctor beg his bread'.

Apple history

According to archaeological research there's evidence that apples were enjoyed by humans as long ago as 6500BC. The apple tree, thought to possibly be the earliest tree to be cultivated, originated in an area between the Caspian and the Black Sea, and is now a familiar sight in many gardens and orchards. Alexander the Great takes the credit for finding dwarfed apples in 300BC in Asia Minor, and the Romans for discovering that apples could be cultivated into sweet-tasting fruits. Many years later apple seeds were introduced to New York (the Big Apple) in the 1600s by early settlers from Europe.

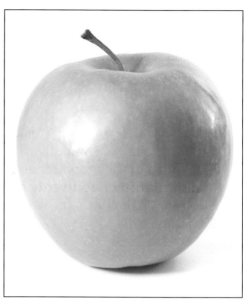

"Keep the doctor away with one of these"

Over the years apples have been prominent in health, mythology and religion. The father of medicine, Hippocrates, is said to have apples as one of his favourite remedies.

In Norse mythology they were offered to the gods to help them achieve eternal youthfulness. Of course in the Garden of Eden Adam is said to have been tempted by Eve to eat an apple such that it became known as the 'forbidden fruit'. Fortunately in modern times we can enjoy apples without suffering any burden of guilt.

Apple remedies

- **Hayfever** – Apples contain quercetin, a flavonoid, which has natural antihistamine effects. Quercetin is thought to stop mast cells releasing histamine, the chemical that triggers allergy symptoms. So eating a couple of apples a day can help to overcome symptoms of hayfever
- **Reflux** – Many people find that eating an apple or drinking a glass of apple juice helps overcome symptoms of heartburn and acid reflux. It's important to seek medical advice if attacks are frequent or persistent
- **Irritated eyes** – Grated apple made into a poultice and placed over the closed affected eye for twenty to thirty minutes helps to treat irritated eyes. Do this once a day for a couple of days. Another option is to peel and slice an overripe apple, place the pulp over closed eye, and hold in place with a bandage
- **Skin irritation** – Cut an apple in half and then rub it against the skin to help soothe the irritation, for example, sunburned skin
- **Tired facial skin** – Mix three tablespoons of apple juice with three tablespoons of lemon juice. Soak a cotton wool ball in the mixture and apply to face

- **Dry cough** – Steam an apple, add two tablespoons of honey, mix together and consume. This helps to relieve a dry tickly cough and may help clear mucus
- **Cleaning teeth and gums** – Eaten raw an apple cleans the teeth and gives the gums a good massage

---

Fighting diarrhoea

Diarrhoea is a common and unpleasant problem. To ease diarrhoea grate a raw unpeeled apple, place on a plate or in a dish for fifteen to twenty minutes until it turns brown and oxidised. Then eat the browned apple, which can be mixed with banana if desired. It is the pectin in apple that helps to bind bowel motions and so stop the diarrhoea.

Conclusion

An apple a day, what more can be said about this most practical and nutritious fruit? Moreover it comes in its own natural wrapping with minimal waste. One medium-sized apple provides one of the UK recommended daily five portions of fruit and vegetables contributing fibre, vitamins, and some minerals to our diet.

A very versatile fruit to have around the home it is a great snack, often one part of a packed lunch, and can be used for a variety of foods and drinks. As we've seen it can be put to very good use in treating minor ailments.

There's a variety to suit all tastes, so make sure there are always apples in your fruit bowl.

ARNICA

The athlete's friend, that's arnica. You don't have to be an athlete though to benefit from this cheerful member of the daisy family. Anyone can benefit when on the receiving end of bumps and knocks. More and more in the playground or on the sportsfield you'll hear the call, 'arnica, please'. It's a good idea to have it with you so that call can be answered.

About arnica

Arnica has now reached a position in healthcare where in my mind, and in the mind of many others, it's mainstream. No longer is it the case that mention of the word 'arnica' brings raised eyebrows and quizzical expressions. Scientific research is quite supportive of arnica, although it's by no means clear-cut. However, the fact that many athletes are said to reach for the arnica when they've overdone it or when suffering an injury has helped to position arnica in a place where there's a relative lack of controversy surrounding it, unlike other therapies. It's certainly something that I always have in my first-aid kit, because you never know when you're going to need it, particularly if you have adventurous children.

Arnica has anti-inflammatory benefits, making it very useful for treating aching and sore muscles. It can be found in many different products – cream, ointment, gel, and spray – the flower heads or plant roots being used. The flower can be made into a poultice by soaking in water that can then be applied to the skin to bring relief. Often tinctures are used, where the herb is mixed with alcohol, in a compress or mouthwash, for example. Arnica also has some anti-microbial and anti-fungal properties making it useful in treating minor skin complaints such as boils.

Did you know?
Arnica plants can be used to freshen the air, since when rubbed their leaves have a strong pine-sage aroma.

Arnica history

Arnica has a long track record of being used to treat bumps and bruises by physicians who made use of its leaves and roots. It's reported that those involved in adventure, for example mountain climbers and explorers, would chew the fresh plant to ease muscle aches and treat the inevitable bruising they would suffer as a consequence of their activities. Because of arnica's anti-microbial properties it was also used to treat gunshot wounds.

Early settlers used alcohol-based tinctures to improve circulation and to treat sore throats

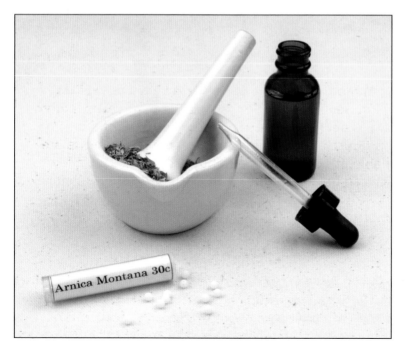

"Arnica continues to be a popular remedy"

and in the Sixteenth Century the German writer Goethe was said to have drunk arnica tea to treat the angina chest pains he suffered. The leaves are also reported to have been smoked.

In years gone by arnica was consumed being believed to help a number of conditions, for example, to improve circulation. However, consumption of arnica is no longer recommended as it is poisonous and can irritate the stomach and intestine causing vomiting, diarrhoea, and abdominal pain. It may also cause difficulty breathing, and possibly death. Some homeopathic practitioners recommend its use, but if being considered for consumption this should always be under close and experienced medical supervision.

Arnica remedies

- **Joint stiffness** – Applying a tincture of arnica to the affected joint or joints can help to relieve stiffness. This can be applied with a compress or poultice and fixed to the joint with a bandage and left for fifteen to twenty minutes
- **Acne** – Ready-made arnica cream can be applied to acne spots making use of the anti-inflammatory and anti-microbial properties of arnica. Alternatively boil arnica flowers in water for five to ten minutes, strain the liquid and then apply to the acne spot using cotton wool once the liquid is at a temperature that the skin can tolerate
- **Muscle sprains** – A cold compress of arnica or a warm poultice applied to the affected muscle can help to reduce swelling, and ease soreness
- **Athlete's foot** – Arnica is believed to have anti-fungal properties so can be used to treat fungal infections of the skin, such as athlete's foot
- **Mouth ulcers** – The anti-inflammatory benefits of arnica can be put to good use in relieving painful mouth ulcers. Using a few drops of arnica in warm water rinse the mouth with the solution as needed, then spit out, do not swallow

Fighting bruises
The most common use for arnica is for treating bruises. This benefit has been used for centuries and has recently become more mainstream as people increasingly recognise its usefulness. Commercial products, for example creams, containing arnica are widely available. It's also possible to buy arnica tincture, a few drops of which can be added to a clean cloth or dressing to make a compress that is then applied to the bruised area of the body.

Conclusion

A member of the daisy family, like its other relatives it's a cheerful-looking flower that in itself is therapeutic. It certainly has the potential to bring much cheer to those who have suffered at the hand of injury in one way or another.

Nowadays it's easy to have arnica to hand when needed because its popularity has meant arnica-containing products are readily available. Whether you're an athlete or simply someone like me who from time to time feels the sudden pain of an accidental bump or knock, arnica really can come to the rescue, and provide a therapeutic 'there, there, there'.

WARNING:
Arnica can be used to treat a number of minor skin complaints effectively, however, it should not be used on broken skin. Doing so may cause skin irritation and a rash.

It's not advisable to take arnica by mouth, unless under strict supervision of a healthcare professional, as it can be poisonous.

BANANAS

As I sit writing this chapter I'm smiling. Why? Because on my desk in front of me is a banana smiling back at me. Comedy has long used the banana to get a laugh, from the person slipping on a banana peel to a banana being stuck in a car's exhaust to immobilise it. I used to enjoy watching the antics of the *Banana Splits* on television, and still enjoy making and eating banana split ice cream sundaes from time to time, which seem to become more elaborate each time I make one. Common minor ailments may not be a laughing matter, but have a banana to hand and you too could be laughing.

About bananas

Elongated, curved, and their being bright yellow lifts the mood. You're bound to have noticed this? If not, give it a try. Moreover, they are a good source of the chemical tryptophan that is converted in the body to the feel-good hormone serotonin. So their cheerful appearance and contents can help us feel good in ourselves.

A rich source of fibre they are one of the first things recommended when someone is suffering with varying degrees of constipation, which just so you know, doesn't only mean not going at all. Medically-speaking someone is considered constipated if they are going less frequently, producing less, and having to put in more effort to go than they usually would. The fibre helps the bowel to function properly, and in fact when someone is suffering with diarrhoea bananas can help too, by binding. Bananas are also packed with vitamins, notably A, the B vitamins and some vitamin C. Also included in this ready-made snack that comes in its own biodegradable wrapper are calcium, magnesium, and a little zinc and iron.

But it's as a dietary energy source that bananas are possibly most well known. Many times you'll see tennis stars enjoying a quick banana in between games. Bananas are rich in carbohydrates that not only provide a rapid burst of energy but also provide a slightly prolonged supply of energy too. In fact, some schools are now encouraging students to eat a banana before sitting exams as research has shown that eating bananas helps to keep students alert.

And in these worrying times of fuel shortage in the future the banana may hold the key to providing not only our body with energy but our homes too. Engineers in Australia have worked out a way to use rotting bananas to make household electrical power, not that you'd want to let a banana rot.

Did you know?

In the year 2000 the Food and Drugs Administration (FDA) in America approved a new health claim that allows potassium-rich and sodium-low foods to make the health claim that their foods may help reduce the risk of high blood pressure and the risk of stroke. Bananas are a very rich source of potassium, which helps lower blood pressure, and fulfil the necessary criteria. They now have established themselves as an important member of the team of measures available to help lessen the risk of these potentially fatal medical conditions.

Banana history

It's suspected by some experts that the banana may have actually been the Earth's first fruit. It can be traced back as far as the Sixth Century BC where it is mentioned in the writings of Buddhist Pali. The banana is believed to originate in Malaysia, from where it travelled to India. It was there that Alexander the Great enjoyed the pleasures of the banana and subse-

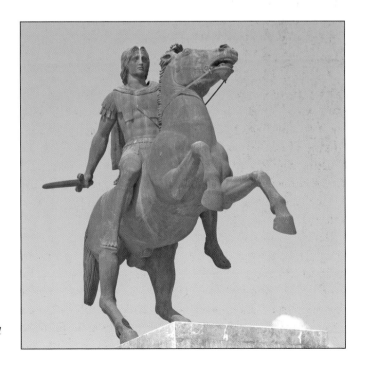

"He knew what the banana had to offer"

quently made it possible for us to enjoy it too, as he is credited with having brought the banana to the Western World.

Interestingly, many years ago in the 1870s when bananas first arrived in North America instructions about how to eat a banana appeared in the Domestic Cyclopaedia of Practical Information stating, 'Bananas are eaten raw, either alone or cut in slices with sugar and cream, or wine and orange juice. They are also roasted, fried, or boiled, and are made into fritter, preserves, and marmalades.' I guess when faced with a new food it's important to know what to do with it, although in my experience experimentation is usually fruitful.

Banana remedies

- **Constipation** – Eat a banana raw or mash first and then eat. If desired it can be liquidised if this makes it easier to consume
- **Bruises and sore skin** – Rub the inside of a banana peel against the sore area of skin, or against insect bites and stings, to reduce uncomfortable inflammation and swelling. For bruises apply the inside of the peel against the bruise, bandage this in place, and leave for twelve to twenty-four hours
- **Heartburn** – Bananas are a natural antacid so eating one can relieve uncomfortable indigestion and heartburn. Bananas also help increase production of protective stomach-lining mucus. Always seek medical advice if these symptoms are frequent or recur
- **Hangovers** – Carbohydrates in bananas help to raise depleted sugar levels, which is what causes the woozy sensations of a hangover
- **Headaches** – Make a poultice of ripe banana peel and place against the sore area of the head

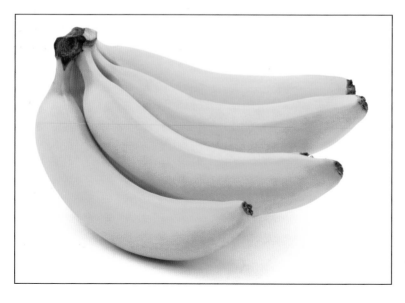

"Goodness inside and out"

- **Morning sickness** – Bananas are a food that is unlikely to upset an upset stomach further and help to raise low blood sugar levels. In this way they can help to overcome morning sickness suffered by women in pregnancy, a feeling that is not only very unpleasant but also can happen at any time of the day, not just in the morning

Fighting verrucas and warts

For many years people have used bananas, the peel to be precise, to treat verrucas and warts. In fact, in my experience as a doctor even after conventional treatments have failed to treat stubborn verrucas the banana peel remedy often does the trick. Some research supports the use of banana peel to treat verrucas and warts. The mucilage within the peel is thought to be the beneficial component. Cut a piece of the skin large enough to cover the wart, tape it securely in place (inner side of the peel against the verruca or wart) and leave overnight. Do this each evening until the verruca or wart disappears.

Conclusion

If you're asked, 'what's your favourite food?' it's not always easy to answer is it? When I'm asked this question I usually offer up an answer, that's quickly followed with, 'well, actually I also like. . .', and this continues until I've named my 'Top Ten' or I've had to admit that I don't have a favourite food – I like lots of food! However, if anyone asks what my favourite fruit is, that's easy. It's the banana.

For as long as I can remember I've enjoyed banana sandwiches, sliced banana in custard, and of course, just a banana alone. Along with tomato soup it's a food I can remember as a child being happy to eat when unwell – I didn't know then that it can help settle a queasy stomach.

So make sure that you don't find yourself in the same situation as those singing the famous folk song written by Frank Silver and Irving Cohn who exclaimed, 'Yes! We have no bananas. We have no bananas today!'

BASIL

Basil is a wonderful herb known to most of us for its flavour. It's also known as the bringer of good luck and fortune, and is considered a king amongst herbs. Basil is thought to be able to calm down inflammation and see off infections too. So be sure to have some basil in your kitchen and in addition to some excellent flavour, and good luck, you will enjoy a good remedy for minor health complaints.

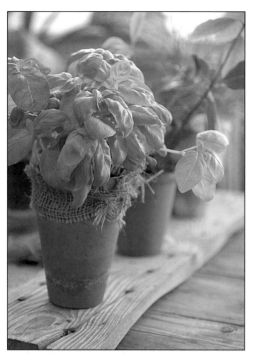

"The bringer of good fortune"

About Basil

Basil is often said to be the king of herbs. In fact, the word basil is derived from the Greek word 'basileus' meaning 'king' or 'basilikon' meaning 'royalty'. This emphasises how over the years basil has been held in high regard by those who have known it and it still holds this superior position in kitchens around the globe.

A member of the mint family, basil is a well-known herb commonly used in everyday cooking. Best used fresh it's added towards the end of cooking to maintain its flavour which would otherwise be destroyed by cooking. It is one of the main ingredients of pesto and is often added to soups. Basil may also be used alongside fruit in sauces and jams.

Basil is a rich source of antioxidant substances, such as flavonoids, and is believed to help keep the heart and circulation healthy and to protect against DNA damage. Basil also contains magnesium which helps keep heart rhythm steady, keeps bones strong, and helps muscles and nerves to function properly. Other compounds found in basil, volatile oils, have been found in scientific studies to be able to inhibit the growth of bacteria. Basil is a good source of vitamins C and A, and calcium. It also contains iron, potassium, and magnesium.

However, basil wasn't always held in such high regard. It was believed to be a symbol of lunacy and malice by the Greeks and Romans. Perhaps this is partly why the well-known comedy character Basil Fawlty (played by the actor John Cleese) in the legendary television show *Fawlty Towers* got his name!

Did you know?

Basil was often given to new homeowners to wish them luck, and to this day a sprig of basil may be placed in a business cash register to bring success and prosperity. Italian women who placed a pot of basil outside their homes were said to be receptive to lovers.

Basil history

There are more than sixty varieties of basil, scientifically called *Ocimum basilicum*. Although traditionally associated with Italian cooking basil actually originated in the Far East where it is still a popular addition to many dishes.

Basil has long been held in a position of high regard representing all things good. In India it is seen as sacred to the Gods and is a symbol of hospitality. Its association with love has great prominence. In parts of Europe, for example, basil is seen as a symbol of love, and if a woman gave a man a sprig of basil it was believed he would love her. If two lovers put basil leaves into a fire what happened to the leaves would predict what would happen in their relationship. Leaves immediately consumed meant they would be happy together, leaves that crackled and flew apart meant things were unlikely to proceed well.

Basil remedies

- **Sore gums** – The soothing benefits of basil can help relieve discomfort through its anti-inflammatory effects. Make a decoction or infusion of basil leaves with boiling water. Allow to cool and then rinse around mouth before either spitting out or swallowing the liquid
- **Sore throat** – The anti-inflammatory, antibacterial, and antiviral properties of basil can help to ease a sore throat, and also coughs and colds. Make a decoction of basil leaves by mashing the leaves and then boiling these in water. Ginger and honey can be added if desired. Allow to cool and then drink
- **Motion sickness** – An infusion of basil can help to ease symptoms of nausea and travel sickness because of its antispasmodic properties. Make an infusion of basil in boiling water, allow to cool, and then drink
- **Stings and minor wounds** – Basil tincture can be used to ease the discomfort of stings and minor wounds. Dilute tincture in water in a ratio of 1:5 and apply with a compress to affected area of skin
- **Digestive problems** – As a member of the mint family it can aid digestion. An infusion of basil consumed after a meal helps to relieve any bloating or discomfort that may have arisen due to overindulgence
- **Aches and pains** – Basil contains oil called eugenol that blocks the effects of an enzyme in the body called cyclo-oxygenase, which would normally trigger inflammation and pain. In this way the oil works in a similar way to conventional anti-inflammatory drugs. Some people find that consuming basil helps relieve symptoms of arthritis

Fighting mouth ulcers

For mouth ulcers placing a basil leaf against the ulcer and keeping it there for as long as possible can ease pain. Alternatively make a decoction or an infusion of basil leaves in boiling water, allow to cool, and then rinse around the mouth before spitting out or swallowing the liquid.

Conclusion

Used a great deal in cooking to achieve a flavourful dish basil can also help inhibit the growth of bacteria on foods that are not cooked, such as salads. This doesn't mean that when preparing a salad adding basil is an alternative to washing the salad, it simply offers an additional potential protective benefit.

I remember growing up watching the BBC television children's programme *The Herbs* and being fascinated by 'Sir Basil – the King of the herbs' because of the deerstalker he wore. I seem to recall he was a little absent-minded. Well, basil is certainly a worthy contender for the title of 'King of the herbs' and is obviously a handy herb to have around the home. Unlike the character Basil Fawlty, played by the actor John Cleese in the television show *Fawlty Towers* who's stock retort to any request from his wife was an irritated 'Yes, dear', the herb basil we all know and love is all too happy to help out when called upon.

BAY LEAF

Bay leaf is a real winner in and around the home, and for centuries has been regarded as the symbol of success. Worn around the head or the neck of those recognised as champions we too can utilise and celebrate its uses. Simply put, allow bay leaf to spoil you and you will definitely be the recipient of the spoils when treating minor ailments.

About bay leaf

The bay leaf that we know so well and use in cooking is the dried leaf of the bay laurel tree, botanically called *Laurus nobililis*. It is also known as bay laurel, sweet laurel or sweet bay – the name 'bay' coming from the Anglo-Saxon meaning crown. So you can see a theme developing here, as you'll see later on, that bay leaf is truly a superior and respected herb that reflects winners and success.

Having originated in Asia Minor it's now grown throughout the Mediterranean. There are two main types of bay leaf, the Californian bay leaf with its stronger flavour, and the Mediterranean bay leaf. Of course it's in cooking that bay leaf is most commonly used to add its unique strong aroma and spicy flavour to sauces and soups, for instance. Bay leaves are also used to flavour stews, and meat and fish dishes.

But there is another use for bay leaves in the kitchen. A year or so ago I was astonished to find dried bay leaves in one of my kitchen cupboards. Initially I thought nothing of it, and simply accepted that they had been misplaced by accident. After all, my mother-in-law who always travels with a selection of her favourite herbs and spices had recently been holidaying with us and during this stay our kitchen's selection of cooking ingredients had increased exponentially, as it always does when she's here – she takes over the kitchen as she loves to cook, and I love her cooking (and her, I should add), so everyone's happy.

It was only when I was faced with these leaves in every cupboard that I started to get suspicious. A gentle enquiry revealed the purpose. Bay leaves keep insects away. For years people have put them in bags of flour, rice, cereal, and boxed cooking ingredients, for example, before modern day sealed containers became available, to keep bugs away. Clearly for many people this practice continues!

Here's an important warning when using bay leaves. Always remember to remove the leaf before serving dishes where it's been used. There are medical reports of the leaf causing damage to the gullet when swallowed and also becoming stuck in the gullet causing a blockage.

Did you know?
Bay leaves are an excellent defence against attack from insects in and around the house. Put a few bay leaves in cupboards to keep these free of invading creatures.

Bay leaf history

The bay tree and its leaves have a most fascinating history, and throughout the ages have been associated with success.

Legend has it that Apollo (god of prophecy, healing and poetry) fell in love with Daphne but his love was unrequited. As she fled from him she was transformed, or some say transformed herself, into a bay tree. From that day Apollo wore a wreath of laurel leaves around his head, it is said to protect himself from the forces of evil but it may well have been as an act of affection ensuring she was always near to him.

Emperors and victorious Ancient Greek and Roman athletes and soldiers, and other heroes, were crowned with wreaths of laurel to celebrate and honour their success. This tradition continues to this day, notably with triumphant Grand Prix race winners. Scholars are also rewarded. The title of poet laureate being given to the poet of the British Royal Household, and students who successfully complete their period of study receive their baccalaureate.

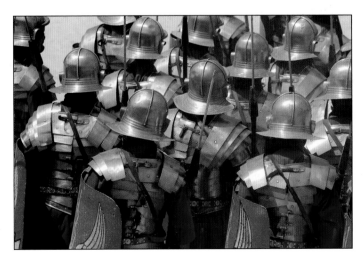

"Victorious return"

For many years bay leaves were believed to ward off evil and bring good fortune. It's not difficult to understand why this might have been since the wreath of leaves was offered to those who had succeeded in their endeavours and doctors wore similar wreaths upon their heads following in the Greek beliefs that bay leaves were a universal cure-all.

Bay leaf remedies

- **Chest complaints** – Make a poultice of bay leaves after boiling these in water. When cool enough apply directly to the chest and cover with a dry cloth. Leave for up to thirty minutes. This can also be used to ease a sore throat by applying to the outside of the throat
- **Promotes sweating** – Make an infusion of bay leaves, allow to cool to a comfortable drinking temperature, and then drink. This can help to encourage sweating when an infection is present
- **Stomach upset** – An infusion of bay leaves taken once or twice a day can help to settle an upset stomach, relieve excessive wind and belching, and help the gut to function properly
- **Dandruff** – Crumble half a dozen bay leaves and add these to boiling water. Allow this to brew for thirty minutes, strain and put into a container to cool. Rinse hair with water, massage the bay tea into the hair, wait a few minutes and repeat with more bay tea. Leave for about one hour then rinse out
- **Stress** – Place bay leaves, camomile, and bergamot into a cloth bag and rest head on this to help reduce stress and induce good sleep

Fighting sore muscles and joints

Bay leaves have long been used to ease the discomfort and pain of swollen and inflamed muscles and joints. A simple approach to this is to soak in a hot bath with loose bay leaves added, or leaves tied up in a small muslin cloth and left in the water. This cloth bag has an added advantage in that you can use it to gently rub against the sore area. Alternatively, soaking the muslin bag in hot water, allowing it to cool, and then applying it to the sore area provides benefit without having to have a bath, getting into which can be challenging for someone with arthritis.

Another way of gaining the benefits for sore muscles and joints is to heat a handful of bay leaves in olive oil for fifteen to twenty minutes and then allow to simmer for a further ten minutes. Strain the oil, and rub against the affected area once cool enough to do so.

Conclusion

It's no wonder wreaths of laurel have symbolised, and continue to symbolise, success because bay leaves really are an all-round winner. From keeping insects from spoiling food ingredients, through helping to provide wonderful flavour to dishes, to helping us to battle with everyday health complaints, bay leaves deserve their accolade.

For me I think Nicholas Culpepper summed it up when in 1653 he wrote about the curative powers of bay leaves, stating, 'Neither witch nor devil, thunder nor lightening will hurt a man where a bay tree is.' Nowadays you don't have to have a bay tree, as my wonderful mother-in-law showed me, a handful of bay leaves will do. Come to think of it, we haven't been troubled by ants for a while …

BICARBONATE OF SODA

This simple but fantastic substance goes by many different names and has even more beneficial uses. Chemists know it as sodium bicarbonate ($NaHCO_3$), cooks know it as baking soda, and my mum simply calls it 'bicarb'. You may also know it as bicarbonate of soda, bread soda, cooking soda, bicarb soda, or sodium hydrogencarbonate. Take a look in your kitchen cupboard, I'll be astounded if you don't have any because it's a basic cooking ingredient that no kitchen should be without.

About Bicarbonate of Soda

This white powder is best known for its use in cooking. I feel I may be teaching Grandma to suck eggs here, but for those of you not in the know, it's a leavening agent used to get

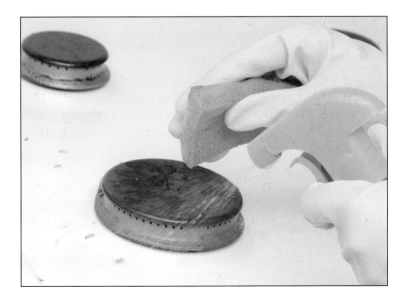

"A helping hand"

breads and cakes to rise, and thus spare the blushes of those of us whose cooking may be witnessed and experienced by others. Bicarbonate of soda is able to do this because it reacts with acidic components in foods resulting in the production of carbon dioxide gas, which fills the food and lifts it. I found out how effective it is years ago when a very good friend of mine added too much to a Yorkshire pudding mixture. The pudding rose beautifully but so much we had to scrape it off the roof of the oven. He blamed the baking soda for this monstrous erection and, as a trusted friend, who am I to doubt him?

As a cleaning agent, bicarbonate of soda will turn its hand to most things. Stains from mattresses, cups and pans, baths and chrome fittings can all be eliminated. Those of us who have a loving relationship with our cars find that chrome fixtures clean up beautifully. If face-cloths and dishcloths smell a little aged, but you're not ready to part company with them, these can be freshened up nicely with bicarbonate of soda.

The downside of cooking for me is not only when the recipe doesn't come out right, it's also the fact that an inevitable consequence is having to clean and tidy up afterwards. A chore I dislike, and I know others dislike too, is having to clean a greasy oven. Bicarbonate of soda can help here as well. Once the oven has been cleaned, applying a paste of water and bicarb to its inside with a brush means it will be easier to clean next time round as the debris will come away with ease.

Did you know?

Bicarbonate can be used to remove mould from a shower curtain. This is helpful from a bathroom aesthetics point of view, but also helpful for those who suffer with mould-related allergies. Mix with water to make a paste of water and bicarbonate of soda, apply to the shower curtain, and leave until dry. Then wash the curtain and the mould should disappear.

Bicarbonate of soda remedies

- **Cystitis** – Drinking half a teaspoon of bicarbonate of soda dissolved in water makes urine less acidic and, consequently helps relieve irritation
- **Earwax** – Drops of bicarbonate of soda dissolved in water can be used to soften hard earwax. This helps wax to naturally fall out of the ear, as it does normally during the day and night, and helps the effectiveness of ear syringing when needed
- **Indigestion / heartburn** – Neutralises the stomach acid responsible for causing indigestion and heartburn. Bicarbonate of soda is found in some commercial antacids. Mix a teaspoon of it into warm water and drink
- **Insect bites and stings** – Bee sting venom is acidic so can be neutralised with bicarbonate of soda once the sting is removed. This will reduce the pain. Make a paste of bicarbonate of soda and water, spread it over the stung area, and leave for five to ten minutes

"Always have a spoonful to hand"

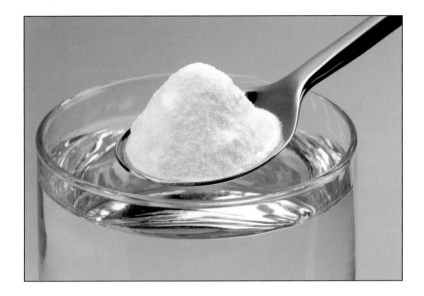

- **Itchy rashes** e.g. poison ivy, bacterial infection, chickenpox, sunburn – Adding bicarbonate of soda to bath water and bathing is good for chickenpox and sunburn where the skin irritation is likely to be widespread. Soaking itchy feet in warm water with some added, or applying a solution of it mixed with water to the itchy part of the body can help relieve the itching
- **Acne** – Some people report an improvement in their acne and skin after applying a paste of bicarbonate of soda and water to their face

Fighting body odour

Bicarbonate of soda absorbs sweat, liquid, and other substances that contribute to the embarrassing and pungent odours that emanate from the armpits, feet, and groin. Not only can it be used to neutralise these odours, it can also be used to remove body odour smells and stains from clothing that contribute to persistent body odours. A simple way to make use of bicarbonate of soda is to dust some powder onto the skin with a powder puff.

Conclusion

The list of uses for bicarbonate of soda stretches much further than its use as a raising agent. Yes, it's very useful when cooking, but it's also extremely useful for relieving health complaints. Moreover, when stubborn stains are a problem, bicarb can help out here too, useful when dealing with the aftermath of cooking.

Bicarbonate of soda should be in everyone's home. In fact, an aunt of mine always has some in her wash-bag so, if she runs into problems when travelling, she always has some available.

Many years ago, a well-known credit card company's slogan was 'Don't leave home without it'. They might as well have been talking about bicarbonate of soda.

BROWN SUGAR

The Rolling Stones' song *Brown Sugar* is one that always gets me moving, and makes me feel good. It's conducive to rocking the shoulders and nodding the head. But at the moment it's causing me a problem. It's become stuck in my head whilst researching this chapter, making it hard for me to concentrate. So forgive me if this chapter needs a little sugar to digest. Please bear with me and you'll see how brown sugar can be a real sweet way of treating some minor ailments.

About brown sugar

Brown sugar gets its distinctive colour from the fact that it contains molasses, commonly known as treacle, the by-product of processing sugar beet or sugar cane into sugar. Depending upon the concentration of these the sugar may at one end of the scale be light in colour and at the other end of the scale be much darker in colour. So whether a sugar is white, or a shade of brown, is down to just how much of the final product is molasses.

I find it fascinating that when manufacturing brown sugar many producers simply add molasses to refined white sugar. This helps them to manage the ratio of sugar crystals to molasses, and also helps with costs. Generally speaking the molasses come from sugar cane, but can also come from sugar beet.

Something you're bound to have noticed is that brown sugar has an irritating habit of hardening. You can be just about to set a gentle flow of brown sugar into motion when plop, ungracefully out falls a solid lump of the stuff. It's because the brown sugar has lost its moisture, which has evaporated, that this occurs. To avoid this nuisance brown sugar is best kept in an air-tight container, or in the original plastic bag it came in.

But what if it's in solid lumps and you have your most fault-searching family member or friend visiting? Well, place a slice of apple or a damp paper towel into a sealed jar containing the brown sugar, leave overnight, and that should sort out the problem. If time is of the essence, pop the

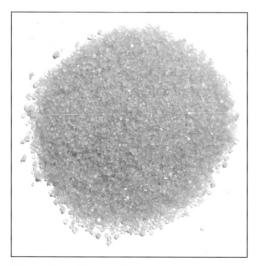

"You make me feel so good"

sugar into the microwave, or on a low heat on the stove for a couple of minutes and then serve immediately.

Did you know?

You can make your own brown sugar at home by simply adding molasses to everyday household refined granulated white sugar. In fact, it's possible to achieve any desired colour in this way. I once heard of someone who was, shall we say rather particular with appearances, and went to great lengths to ensure that the brown sugar served with coffee blended well with the colour of the coffee pot, cups, and the tray on which these were placed.

Brown sugar history

Sugar itself has been around for centuries and is thought to have originated in the South Pacific approximately eight thousand years ago. The journey of sugar to the rest of the world was facilitated by Arabs who arrived in Spain introducing sugar to Europe. As with a number of foods it was Christopher Columbus who was responsible for transporting the sugar cane plant to the Caribbean, where it still continues to be a very popular and economic product.

The process of pressing out the juice from sugar cane and then boiling this juice into crystals of sugar is thought to have begun around 500BC in India. In days gone by brown sugar was created by simply leaving some molasses in, creating semi-refined sugar. Modern day practice has changed somewhat in that now the molasses are removed to make refined white sugar, and molasses added back to achieve the desired ratio and colour. The darker the colour the stronger is the taste.

When the refined white sugar industry took off brown sugar came under attack from those involved in the industry. In the late 1800s they tried to turn people off brown sugar using a smear campaign with photographs showing harmless but nasty looking microbes living in brown sugar.

It's the water in the molasses that gives brown sugar its characteristic fluffiness and why when this evaporates it forms into hard lumps. Before modern sealed containers became available it was noted that much as sugar may have started off its journey as loose granules, on arrival it was often solid and 'brick-like' in its consistency. This meant that cooks had to literally scrap or grate sugar by hand. Thomas Edison came up with the idea of shipping brown sugar in heavily waxed paper, but it was the cooks themselves who thought of including a slice of apple to try and maintain the sugar's moisture content and so prevent hardening.

Brown sugar remedies

- **Menstrual cramps** – A popular Chinese remedy brown sugar is added to ginger – a natural painkiller – tea and a cup consumed a couple of times a day. The nutrients in brown sugar are said to tranquilise the nervous system and so also relieve pain
- **Coughs and colds** – Brown sugar can be added to a mixture of warm water and lemon juice to help soothe a tickly cough and sore throat. Another way of making use of brown sugar is to add it between layers of sliced raw onions in a bowl, and then use the resulting juice as a cough medicine
- **Hiccups** – Eating a spoonful of brown sugar may help by synchronising the nerves that regulate breathing
- **Bruises** – Immediately a bruise begins to appear spread molasses on brown paper and apply to the bruise
- **Rough skin** – Brown sugar granules act as a very good exfoliant and moisturiser for rough skin. First soak the skin in plain warm water, then taking a handful of brown sugar gently rub against the skin. Then wash the skin again and moisturise. Alternatively, a mixture of olive or sesame oil, and brown sugar can be used
- **Diarrhoea / constipation** – Some people find that drinking a solution of one to two teaspoons of brown sugar in warm water helps to either relieve diarrhoea or relieve constipation as needed

Fighting wounds

Sugar has been used to treat wounds for centuries as it dries the wound helping to prevent bacterial growth. It is also an excellent disinfectant helping to kill infecting organisms and speed healing. Around the home brown sugar can be used to help treat minor cuts and burns. Firstly, ensure the wound is clean and then sprinkle the wound lightly with brown sugar. It can help to smear petroleum jelly around the wound to hold the grains of sugar in place and then protect with a clean dressing. Repeat this process once or twice daily. It goes without saying that for major wounds including large or blistering burns and deep cuts, particularly if stopping bleeding is a problem, urgent medical advice should be sought.

Conclusion

OK, so I've finally managed to get the tune out of my head, which is a relief because I actually enjoy it and don't want my future pleasure from it to be diminished. The fluffy brown granules, however, should never be absent from the home. They are best kept in an air-tight container so they'll be ready to assist you in overcoming a number of minor ailments.

Talking of minor ailments, be sure to have some molasses and white sugar available too, in case for some reason you run out of or simply don't have any brown sugar around. You never know when you might need some for yourself, or when a friend is round for a chat and says, 'Oh, you haven't got any brown sugar, have you?' For me though now, it's time for a coffee break.

CABBAGE

This wonderful green leaf vegetable is very popular amongst adults, but less so amongst children. Those amongst us who are parents know all too well how children often turn their nose up when confronted with boiled cabbage. In time they'll learn how good cabbage is for a healthy body as it's a rich source of health promoting antioxidants. In the meantime let's learn about how cabbage can relieve common complaints.

About Cabbage

It's interesting how my views about cabbage have been influenced by those around me. I suppose it's similar for many people. I remember growing up and my grandmother often saying to my brother and me, 'Eat up your cabbage. It'll make your hair curly.' This didn't inspire us to eat it as neither of us wanted curly hair. If children at school said 'ugh' to cabbage, the rest of us were likely to follow suit. In more recent times an explosion of wind is often soon followed by a grin and the remark, 'that'll be the cabbage'.

My first introduction to the health benefits of cabbage was when I was embarking on my career in general practice. I learned how cabbage could be put to good use to relieve discomfort. Our practice nurse asked me to review one of our patients who had recently given birth and had uncomfortable breasts. I couldn't help noticing her bra packed with cabbage leaves,

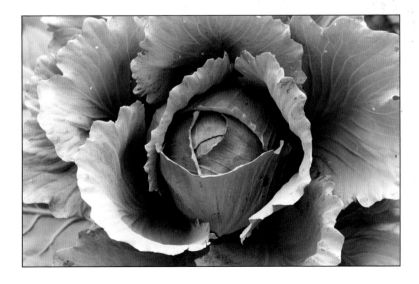

but tried not to stare or make any comment. After all, people do the strangest things and who am I to judge. Anyway, it soon became apparent that she had mastitis, was benefitting from the effects of the cabbage leaves, and didn't need any further treatment. And since that day, I've been recommending the same.

Cabbage is classified as a leaf vegetable and is part of the *Cruciferae* family along with Brussels sprouts, cauliflower, and broccoli. Normally the part of the cabbage that's eaten is the immature leaves, or cabbage head. This may be eaten raw often as strips in coleslaw, or cooked either as an accompanying vegetable or as part of a dish such as stews or soups – one of my favourites is corned beef and cabbage. Sauerkraut is made from fermented cabbage and is popular in many parts of Europe, notably Germany. Kimchi is another popular fermented Korean cabbage dish.

A few words of caution. Using cabbage leaves to treat mastitis in breastfeeding women may lessen milk supply so for this reason once relief is achieved cabbage leaves should be removed and used again if discomfort returns. Cabbage contains substances that can affect the functioning of the thyroid gland. For this reason those who have thyroid problems should seek medical advice before changing their usual consumption of cabbage. Boiled cabbage may cause excessive flatulence, as you may know!

Did you know?
Captain James Cook carried sauerkraut on his voyages to prevent his crew from developing scurvy as cabbage is a good source of vitamin C.

Cabbage history

Cabbage is believed to have been grown in Ancient Greek and Roman civilisations, and derived from a leafy wild mustard plant. The word cabbage is a derivation of the French word 'caboche', a colloquial term for 'head'. Celtic wanderers are thought to have brought it to Europe in around 600BC where it became a very popular vegetable not only for food but also for treating a number of health conditions. The familiar and popular Savoy cabbage, with its round head and crinkled leaves and whose name derives from its popularity in the French Savoie Alpine region, is said to have been developed by the Italians.

More recently cabbage has found popularity since it is rich in antioxidants, for example vitamins A and C, and folate, all of which are believed to help keep the heart and circulation healthy. Cabbage consumed as part of a healthy balanced diet may also help since fibre can help to lower cholesterol levels in the blood and consequently protect the heart and circulation. Cabbage may also help to prevent cancer as studies have demonstrated that those who eat lots of cruciferous vegetables have a lower risk of colorectal, prostate, and lung cancers. In one study those eating three or more servings of cruciferous vegetables a week had a forty-four per cent lower risk of prostate cancer.

Cabbage remedies

- **Inflammation** – Cabbage contains an amino acid called glutamine, which can help to reduce inflammation. It also contains omega-3 fatty acids that are anti-inflammatory. Make a paste of raw cabbage, put this in a cabbage leaf and place on or around the affected area
- **Constipation** – Cabbage is a rich source of dietary fibre that can help the gut function properly, help prevent constipation, and help to relieve constipation when consumed as part of a healthy balanced diet
- **Boils** – To relieve the inflammation of a boil apply a fresh cabbage leaf to the boil and secure this in place
- **Tired feet** – Soften two cabbage leaves by blanching then cut out the hard fibres that run through the leaves. Fold or roll up the leaves and place into the arch of the foot. Hold in place with a bandage
- **Peptic ulcer** – Drinking raw cabbage juice has been shown in scientific research to heal ulcers in the stomach and the duodenum (the upper part of the small intestine). A glass of raw cabbage juice consumed four times a day for ten to fourteen days is recommended. **WARNING:** Always seek medical advice before trying this treatment
- **Scurvy** – Cabbage is a good source of vitamin C so can help to prevent scurvy that although uncommon in the UK still occurs around the world
- **Gout** – With a rolling pin crush one or two cabbage leaves after softening in boiling water. Fold in half and then apply to the affected area. This remedy can also be used to relieve headaches by placing the cabbage against the forehead or back of the neck

Fighting mastitis

Mastitis occurs when the breast becomes inflamed, commonly although not exclusively in breastfeeding women.

The effect of cooling or heating plus the release of anti-inflammatory chemicals from cabbage leaves eases discomfort. Chilled cabbage leaves can be placed against the affected breast, most easily achieved by lining the bra cup with the leaves. This has the effect of a cold compress and so relieves swelling and heat in the same way. Leaves can be left for a couple of hours and then replaced a couple of hours later.

Another way is to warm up the leaves first, by blanching them in boiling water, running a hot iron over them, or putting them in a microwave. Heating is believed to help release the anti-inflammatory chemicals from the cabbage leaves. Check that they are not too hot before using. Some people recommend bruising the leaves with a rolling pin first before placing the leaves in the bra to help release the anti-inflammatory chemicals.

Conclusion

Cabbage is a wonderful vegetable that is found in most kitchens. Delicious to eat it should be a fundamental part of a balanced healthy diet.

Cabbage is practical and easy to use to relieve swollen and uncomfortable parts of the body. In addition, when the bowels become a little sluggish, boiled cabbage helps come to the rescue.

As adults we're already aware of the joy of cabbage, and in time most children come to love cabbage too.

CALENDULA

Let's add some colour. This is the call of many a person wandering around a garden centre. And where do we turn first, something bright and cheerful, and usually yellow. And marigolds, or calendula, provide this. In fact they add colour to more than just the environment. They add colour to foods, and when treating minor ailments, to our health too.

About calendula

I've had marigolds in my garden, and in my home, for years. One way or another they seem to come my way. I can't remember ever initiating any of these plants? They've always appeared as gifts from visiting family and friends, or from my neighbour who had a remarkable ability to propagate seeds such that plants would appear in the trays in what I can only describe as a regimented fashion. Looking at the rows of his propagation trays was like watching a miniature botanical version of 'Trooping the Colour', but less tiring. But it wasn't until a number of years ago when I was given a tube of cream containing calendula, and got great use out of it, that I made the connection between the two. So you could say with regard to calendula I was a late developer.

This wonderful member of the daisy family enjoys the botanical name *Calendula officinalis*. The name comes from the Latin kalendae, meaning the first day of the month, believed to have stemmed from the fact that in some parts of the world it blooms every month. We mostly know it as marigold, or pot marigold, which is said to refer to the Virgin Mary or its old English Saxon name 'ymbglidegold', which means it turns with the sun – not surprising since its cheerful colouring like the sun brings warmth, brightness and a cheerful mood.

Its petals are edible and often fresh ones are finely chopped and added to salads, where these add colour. Dried petals, having a more bitter taste, are added to soups and cakes. In fact, it's also added to chicken feed so it can darken the colour of egg yolks.

Calendula has many health benefits, it being antiseptic and anti-inflammatory, and so finds great use in healing many minor skin complaints such as burns and stings. Some research suggests it is helpful for those women with breast cancer undergoing radiation therapy in preventing skin dermatitis, a possible consequence of this treatment. If you'd like some chemistry the petals contain triterpenoid esters that are anti-inflammatory and carotenoids that are antioxidants and also responsible for its wonderful bright colouring. Calendula may well also have antiviral, antibacterial and anti-fungal benefits too.

I have a tube of calendula cream that I always carry with me when out with my family. Calendula really is a first aid item, and with first aid, you need to have it ready. Moreover, extract the sap from the stem by crushing it and its application may help to treat warts, corns, and calluses. Taken internally, as tea or a tincture for example, calendula is thought to help strengthen the circulation and to speed up wound healing, whilst also helping to heal any digestive inflammation.

Did you know?

An infusion of the petals can be used as a rinse to lighten hair. Also, these petals can advise whether you need an umbrella or not since they close up when wet weather is likely to occur. Being from Wales I'm familiar with some people suggesting this and saying if they don't open during the day, then be prepared for stormy weather. This isn't something I've studied, but perhaps in the future I may put this to a scientific test.

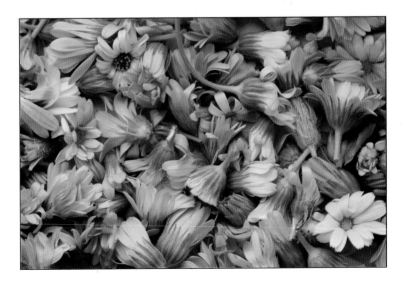

"An abundance of soothing"

Calendula history

Calendula really has been used for a long time. Over the years its bright colouring was believed to help strengthen the heart both physically and mentally by clearing the mind and encouraging happiness. The Egyptians valued calendula as a great healer and rejuvenator. To hang garlands of marigolds over the entrance to the home was believed to prevent evil spirits from entering. Nowadays marigold petals can be found in pot-pourri, where presumably the same benefit may occur – this can certainly add a pleasant aroma to a room.

In Ancient Greek and Roman times it was used for its medicinal properties, and in Indian and Arabic cultures for this too. Adding colour is a theme with calendula and these same cultures used it as a dye for cosmetics, foods and fabrics. In fact its petals have been used to colour foods such as cheese and butter. Its culinary use doesn't stop there with many using its petals as a more economic alternative to saffron, a practice the Romans employed.

Large amounts of calendula are now grown in the former Soviet Union where locally it is known as Russian penicillin.

Calendula remedies

- **Haemorrhoids** – The antiseptic and anti-inflammatory properties can be put to good use in relieving uncomfortable and irritating haemorrhoids, and also painful anal fissures. Calendula can be applied in cream or ointment form. Alternatively make an infusion of calendula leaves and having soaked a clean cloth with this, apply to the affected area. It can be applied as a warm poultice too
- **Minor burns** – Calendula is well recognised as being very effective for treating minor burns, scalds, and sunburn. It's best to have a treatment ready, for example an ointment, to apply as soon as needed
- **Impetigo** – Since calendula has some antibacterial properties these can be put to good use in helping to treat this highly contagious bacterial skin infection. It may be applied using a cream or a compress
- **Cold sores** – Calendula has some antiviral effects so can help to treat uncomfortable cold sores. This can be applied using a tincture on cotton wool
- **Varicose veins** – Drinking a herbal calendula tea, made by infusing the petals, twice daily may help to relieve the symptoms of varicose veins and lessen their appearance
- **Fungal skin infections** – Amongst its many other properties calendula also is thought to have some degree of anti-fungal activity so it can be used to help treat fungal infections. It may be applied to the affected area as a cream or by soaking cotton wool in a cooled infusion

Fighting skin complaints

Calendula is best known for its many benefits in treating minor skin ailments such as pimples and eczema, and those caused by infection or physical damage. Not only is it anti-inflammatory and antiseptic but it is also very soothing. Calendula can be applied as a tincture, poultice, compress, cream or ointment.
The choice is yours.

Conclusion

Ah, marigolds. Even that particular brand of rubber gloves is often yellow, well, in my home they are. Calendula for me is a provider, of colour, of happiness, or relief when minor aliments threaten to reverse all these good things.

We know all too well how giving hands may bring beautiful marigold blooms into a person's life. You can always count on a marigold to deliver the goods and be gratefully received. But as we've seen the benefits reach further than just a gift offering. I'll make sure I remember that next time someone gives me a marigold, or better still, when I'm the one doing the giving.

CAMOMILE

My fondness for this pretty little flower with its white petals and rich yellow centre is far-reaching. Simply gazing at it brightens up my day. But more than this, camomile is one herb that in my experience everyone has something positive to say about, particularly when it comes to helping to deal with minor ailments.

About camomile

My introduction to camomile came a number of years ago when I was becoming interested in the role that non-drug therapies can play in treating illness. I'd heard people talk about camomile tea to relieve stress, so tried it. And for me it seemed to work. Busy and fraught general practice clinics became more manageable, I quickly became less stressed. My research confirmed my more relaxed demeanour shouldn't have come as a surprise. Camomile is an effective calmative after all. It's also got anti-spasmodic and muscle relaxing properties. Eager to share my new found knowledge I suggested camomile tea to a retired female patient who was struggling to find time to fulfil her passion for golf. A few weeks later she told me she was back on the golf course, three times a week, and thanked me for my advice. I've been drinking camomile tea and recommending it ever since, even though in the early days I was teased about this by those around me who no doubt wondered if I'd be shedding my black leather shoes for open-toed sandals and my clean shaved look for a beard.

It's not only as herbal tea that it's recognised. Camomile is also used in cooking, being sprinkled over salads, and used as flavouring in sweets and cakes, for example. It's also used to flavour the alcoholic beverage Benedictine, which I am rather partial to from time to time.

Camomile is a member of the sunflower family, and is classified by botanists into two major varieties – the German variety *Matricaria recutita*, and the Roman variety *Anthemis nobilis*. Camomile has always, and continues to be popular around the world, and especially in Greece. In fact, its name, which may also be spelled chamomile, comes from the Greek words for 'ground' and 'apple'. This is because of its aroma being reminiscent of apples and because it grows close to the ground. Isn't it great when explanations are this straightforward!

Despite it being low to the ground for me it's the botanical names that reinforce the image conjured up when I think of camomile, an image of unassuming nobility. Not just because of the name 'nobilis', but because this neat, compact little flower in the herb world is accepted as a very important member with a long history of use through the ages. One in modern day 'street' language, to offer 'respect'.

Did you know?
In the days before refrigeration became available to prevent meat from spoiling it was immersed in camomile infusion.

Camomile history

Since ancient times camomile has been used and respected. The Ancient Egyptians recognised how it could relieve stress and aid restful sleep when anxiety stood in the way of this. They worshipped this flower, its golden centre being offered to the sun god Ra. Ancient Greeks too made good use of camomile, using it to treat chills and fevers. It's said that the physician Dioscorides prescribed Roman army soldiers camomile to treat disorders of the nervous system and gastrointestinal problems.

In India Ayurvedic medicine uses camomile extensively for its benefits in calming an upset stomach, utilising its effects of stopping and preventing spasms. In Medieval times in Europe camomile continued to be used to treat problems such as insomnia, and also as an alternative to grass for lawns.

Camomile was, and still is, burned as an incense to aid meditation and to bring luck and prosperity. Some people apply camomile oil to their body or keep camomile flowers in their purse or wallet to attract money. Camomile can also be used to clean and lighten hair, and is a useful insect repellent.

Of course its action as a calmative is what camomile is best known for, usually taken as herbal tea. But it also has anti-inflammatory, anti-microbial, and anti-spasmodic effects which can be put to very good use in treating minor ailments.

'Time to relax'

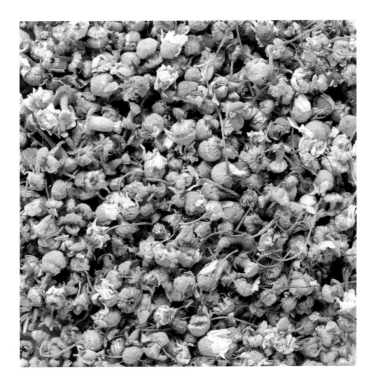

Camomile remedies

- **Insomnia** – This often occurs when something is 'playing on the mind' causing worry and anxiety that in turn prevents the journey into restful sleep. A cup of camomile tea consumed around thirty minutes before bedtime can help relax the mind and body aiding sleep. Alternatively, place a few drops of camomile essential oil onto the pillow or pyjamas

- **Mouth ulcers** – Camomile has anti-inflammatory effects, and may also have anti-microbial effects, that can be put to good use in relieving painful mouth ulcers. Allow a cup of camomile herb tea to cool and then use as a mouth rinse. In can help to make up a container or jug of camomile tea, and store in the fridge ready to use when needed. Cold is best as hot foods and drinks often cause more ulcer discomfort

- **Minor skin irritation** – The mildly antiseptic and anti-inflammatory effects of camomile can help soothe sore and irritated skin. Add a teaspoon of camomile leaves to a cup, and add boiling water. Leave for around five minutes then strain and place the leaves against the affected area, holding in place with a clean dressing. If using a tea bag, apply this to the affected area and leave for twenty to thirty minutes

- **Gut spasms** – Drinking warm camomile tea helps to relieve gut spasm caused by conditions such as irritable bowel syndrome. Some women also gain relief from period pains either by drinking camomile tea or by rubbing camomile essential oil over the lower abdomen and pubic area

Fighting sore eyes

A cup of camomile herbal tea made with a tea bag can be very helpful for soothing sore eyes caused by conditions such as hayfever. After brewing a cup of camomile herb tea, remove the tea bag and allow this to cool until it's at a temperature that can be tolerated and rest it against closed eyes. Drink the tea to gain additional benefit of relieving any stress the sore eyes have caused, that in turn will be exacerbating the eye soreness. This can also be used to relieve everyday tired and puffy eyes.

Conclusion

Camomile, the noble, gentle and kind herb, is how I like to think of it. It will always have a place in my heart, having helped transport me through some tough times in my early days of general practice, and of course, providing me with a positive introduction to how simple things around us can really help to overcome some health ailments.

Experienced gardeners often call camomile the 'Plant Doctor' because many believe it can help ailing plants near it to recover. In medicine for many years camomile has been used to help in a similar way, and in my mind will always be a natural healer that should be always within arm's reach.

CARROTS

Bugs Bunny loves eating carrots and is always seen in the legendary cartoons eating his way through stacks of them. In reality, carrots are loved by everyone; well almost everyone. Their bright orange colour is cheerful and mood-lifting, their many different and sometimes unusual shapes raise a smile and a laugh, which in itself is a great medicine in my mind. And, if that's not enough, carrots are something to have to hand for everyday common complaints.

About carrots

I don't know anyone who doesn't like carrots. This vegetable in my experience is universally loved, and by all ages. Carrots are one vegetable that even children are happy to eat. Is that any surprise? Well no. Crisp and crunchy, tasty, and brightly coloured eaten raw they make the perfect lunch box snack. They're pretty good as a natural after-meal mouth cleanser and freshener too. Carrots are used in many dishes including soups, stews, and curries, accompanying roast lunch, even cake – carrot cake, containing grated carrot, has become very popular over the years.

Delicious, yes. Nutritious, definitely. Carrots are a rich source of antioxidants that neutralise potentially damaging free radicals in the body. Notably carrots are rich in vitamin C, potassium, and dietary fibre. Of course, they are very rich in vitamin A, an antioxidant vitamin that is renowned for its ability to aid good vision.

Carrots can help good vision because they contain beta-carotene that's converted in the body into vitamin A, which is needed and important for healthy eyesight. However, eating carrots does not improve night vision, or daytime vision for that matter, unless a person is vitamin A deficient.

Carrots are a member of the *Umbelliferae* family, whose relatives include parsnips, fennel and dill. There are many varieties of carrots ranging from the very small 'mini' or 'baby' carrots to the much longer carrots we are familiar with. Although everyone knows the shape of carrots, they do come in some peculiar ones too. Certainly some of those I've seen harvested from my family's vegetable garden are hilarious, and others have the shape of little people, sometimes with gender-specific appendages too! In fact, those less embarrassing ones can often be seen on show at village fetes around the country, sometimes even winning prizes for the best unusual shape.

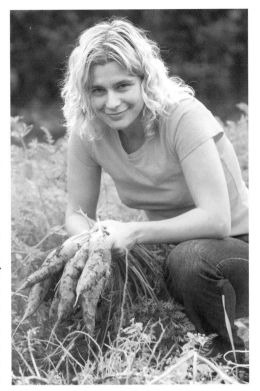
'Pull up some goodness'

Did you know?

The association of carrots with 'seeing in the dark' began in World War 2 and was invented by the British Royal Air Force as a way to explain why suddenly more Nazi bombers were being shot down. The disinformation campaign attributed this success to the pilots consuming carrots, when in fact it was due to a new, and secret, radar system.

Carrot history

Through the ages carrots have been used for all kinds of purposes. It's said that Greek soldiers consumed large quantities of raw carrots to inactivate their bowels whilst travelling within the Trojan horse. The Romans made good use of carrots, calling them purple or white vegetables or carota, both as food and for medicinal purposes believing like the Greeks that carrots were an aphrodisiac. In England the Anglo-Saxons consumed carrot within a drink to ward off insanity and the devil. And during James I reign carrot ferns were worn by women in their hair as a fashionable accessory.

Ask anyone about a carrot and the first thing they are likely to say is it's orange, but this wasn't always the case. Carrots date back centuries, to around 5000BC, in Afghanistan where they are reported as being red, black or deep purple in colour, similar to the purple colouring of eggplants.

In Afghanistan by around 900AD carrots had become yellow in colour where their colour was celebrated because being sun-worshippers people believed eating yellow, and orange, coloured foods instilled a sense of righteousness.

It wasn't until the 1500s though that the orange carrot came into being. Credit for this goes to Dutch scientists who wanted to offer a tribute to the Dutch Royal Family. By cross-breeding pale yellow and red varieties of carrots they successfully created the carrot we know today.

Carrot remedies

- **Fresh breath** – Carrots can help keep the mouth and breath fresh. Eating pieces of crunchy raw carrot can achieve this as it stimulates saliva flow and helps to dislodge food particles from in between the teeth. Alternatively simmer half a dozen carrot tops in water for fifteen to twenty minutes then steep for half an hour. Strain this and keep in the refrigerator to be used as a cool mouth wash
- **Itchy skin** – Apply freshly cut slices of carrot to the itchy areas. Cooled slices may bring even greater relief
- **Warts** – Mix olive oil with grated carrot and apply the mixture to the wart directly or using a clean cloth. Hold in place with a clean dressing for up to an hour or overnight. Repeat this daily until wart has gone
- **Sores** – Using mashed or grated carrots make a poultice with olive oil and apply to the sore, holding in place with a clean dressing for around thirty minutes. Repeat twice daily
- **Burns** – After running cool water over the burn soak a clean dressing in carrot juice and apply to the affected area
- **Dry skin** – Add grated carrots to a tablespoon of natural plain yogurt or cream. Mix to the consistency of a paste and gently rub this over the dry skin areas in a circular motion. This acts as an effective exfoliant and moisturiser. Allow to dry, rinse off with cool water, and pat the skin dry

Fighting blisters

These uncomfortable skin lesions are often caused by the rubbing from poorly fitting footwear. They can be painful but should not be intentionally burst, just allowed to burst of their own accord.

Mashed carrot mixed with a little olive oil or lard can bring relief
when applied to the blister and held in place with a clean
dressing.

Conclusion

There's a lot about carrots that raises eyebrows. There's the hilarious ones my Dad brings
in from his allotment from time to time and if I'm not around to see it in the flesh – a very
appropriate use of the word flesh here when I cast my mind back to the startlingly human
forms his carrots have taken over the years – then I can pretty much guarantee my email inbox
will contain a photo attachment of said creation. But there's also the partial truth partial myth
that carrots help you see better in the dark. Then of course the shocking fact that they weren't
always orange.

One thing's for certain, however, and has over the years been successfully used by many.
The carrot is a useful vegetable to have around when minor health problems arise. Reach
for it and imagine it saying back to you – 'What's up doc?'

CLOVES

It's a funny looking thing the clove. At least I think it is. To me it's always looked like a miniature flower. It's name actually comes from the Latin word 'clavus' meaning nail, which I
guess now I think of it, it does look a bit similar to this. Certainly if you get one in your mouth
without realising it it can cause a specific sensation, not a painful one as a nail would cause,
but distinctive never the less. Here's the good thing though. Sometimes it's good to have
one in the mouth. Truthfully, it is, believe me.

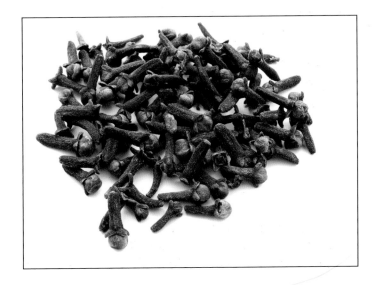

'Surprise soothers'

About Cloves

We all recognise cloves, and their tiny flower-like appearance. In cooking there's a long list of dishes where cloves may be found to add flavour. What springs to my mind are meats studded with cloves, or likewise half an onion studded and added to a soup or stew. These are good because at least this way the cloves are visible, unlike when they are added to an apple pie, for example. On a number of occasions I remember all too well getting caught out by a clove that, like a Ninja warrior, had found its way into my mouth and between my teeth, henceforth reminding me of its powerful flavour.

Nutritionally cloves are a rich source of manganese, fibre, vitamin C, omega-3 fatty acids, calcium and magnesium. Oil of cloves, or clove oil, has been used for many years for its health benefits, notably in dentistry as an analgesic and antiseptic. These effects have been put to good use to relieve toothache and, when dental treatment was being performed, to disinfect root canals. It's the eugenol in the clove oil, extracted from cloves, that is responsible for these benefits, and in fact for the familiar aroma of cloves.

In addition to their use in cuisine cloves are used as a material for incense in Japan and China, and in other countries, for example Indonesia, may be smoked in cigarettes.

Did you know?

Cloves can be used as cosmetics to darken hair. For example, if you're concerned about greying hair mixing ground cloves in ginger root juice and massaging into the hair and scalp will cover these age-revealing hairs up. A well-scorched clove can be stroked onto the eyebrows to darken these.

Clove history

Cloves have been consumed in Asia for over 2000 years, and archaeologists have found cloves in a ceramic vessel in Syria dating back to around 1721BC. For many years cloves were only to be found growing on a few islands of the Spice Islands in Indonesia, now known as the Moluccas. They now can be found in other countries around the world, including Brazil, Mauritius, and the West Indies.

During Roman times the clove was highly prized and in later years heavily traded. The pungent flavour of the clove – that I know very well – was used to good effect to freshen the breath by Chinese courtiers who didn't want to offend their emperor. Chinese physicians used cloves to treat fungal skin infections such as ringworm and athlete's foot, and also indigestion, intestinal parasite infections and diarrhoea. Indian Ayurvedic healers also used cloves to treat digestive and respiratory ailments. Cloves were also used to hide the taste of badly preserved foods.

More recently, until the advent of modern drug treatments, cloves and the essential oil from cloves containing eugenol has been used extensively as an analgesic, anaesthetic, and antiseptic to assist in the treatment of dental complaints, the oil being first extracted from clove buds by the early American Eclectic physicians. Nowadays oil of cloves can often be found added to cough and cold remedies, toothpastes, and mouthwash products.

Clove remedies

- **Bad breath** – Cloves have long been used to overcome the problems of bad breath. Chewing one or two cloves and then spitting these out can help improve the freshness of breath
- **Haemorrhoids** – The anaesthetic effects of clove oil can help to relieve the discomfort of haemorrhoids when applied once or twice a day. It may be easier to mix clove oil with yogurt and apply as a cream. Scientific research has also found that chronic anal fissures can be helped by the application of clove oil in cream
- **Hangover** – The dry mouth, nausea, and muzzy head of a hangover can be helped by chewing on one or two cloves and then spitting these out
- **Stress** – Soaking in a bath with added clove oil can help to relieve stress

Fighting toothache

Without doubt it is in the treatment of dental problems that cloves have shone over the years, a result of the anaesthetic and antiseptic effects of this dried flower bud. To relieve toothache simply chew a clove and roll it around the sore part of the mouth. Alternatively using clove oil dipped onto a cotton bud, apply directly to the sore area.

Conclusion

So there you have it. The little devil that so often as a child and teenager caught me out when I was enjoying home-made apple pie and custard, and to be perfectly honest, cream too, really can have what for me were quite disruptive effects put to very good use. Over the centuries many have benefitted and we can too. So always have cloves and clove oil available and ready, just in case problems arise, as they often do.

COCONUT OIL

Do you have a lovely bunch of coconuts? Don't worry if you don't because what you need is coconut oil and nowadays you don't need to be scrambling up tall palm trees and then toiling over a hot fire to get this. It's readily available in a bottle or other container. If you do have a coconut sitting on your kitchen countertop, it can be put to much more use than just decoration, as it's not only nice to look at.

About coconut oil

Who hasn't enjoyed the challenge of the coconut shy, which is said to have originated in Kingston, Surrey at the annual Pleasure Fair. Some of you may have been smothered in coconut oil when trying to achieve a suntan, in the days when the dangers of suntans were less apparent. Yes, it did smell nice didn't it!

The coconut is a marvellous fruit. It provides water, milk, meat, sugar, and oil and if that isn't enough, it also provides a ready-made cup to drink from. On my first visit to the Caribbean I learned how coconut water is a very popular drink. Small trucks are seen parked along main streets piled high to overflowing with fresh coconuts. People selling them will quickly slice the top off with a machete for you to drink the coconut water, usually through a straw. Not only is coconut water a very refreshing drink it provides a quick burst of energy. The popularity of coconut water has meant that nowadays in the Caribbean, and I'm sure elsewhere, large bottles of it can be found on sale in supermarket refrigeration units. And if you should be snorkelling or scuba diving whilst on holiday rubbing inner coconut husk on the lens of the goggles can prevent these fogging up.

Coconut oil is made in a number of ways. For example, virgin coconut oil is made by quick drying coconut meat then pressing this to extract the oil, or without first drying fresh coconut can be pressed to extract coconut milk that is then separated into oil and water by boiling, fermenting, or other processing. Refined coconut oil is made from the dried coconut meat, called copra, and then deodorised using high heat and bleached through clays to purify it.

Despite its very familiar name the coconut is not actually a nut, it's a seed. In fact, it is the largest seed known. Scientifically it goes by the name *Cocos nucifera* – nucifera means 'nut-bearing'. One reason why the coconut is so popular is because although it takes up to a year to mature, coconut fruit continuously develop on the tree all year round so coconuts are continually available.

Did you know?
You can make your own coconut oil simply at home. Remove coconut meat from coconut, grate this and add water. Squeeze this to make coconut milk then heat until water has gone leaving coconut oil.

Coconut oil history

Who can mistake the hairy brown nut with its three eye-like indentations that so much resembles a friendly head. Because of these features it was called 'coco', meaning 'monkey face', by the early Spanish explorers.

The coconut was first cultivated in the Pacific where to this day it is still known as 'The

"Something for everyone"

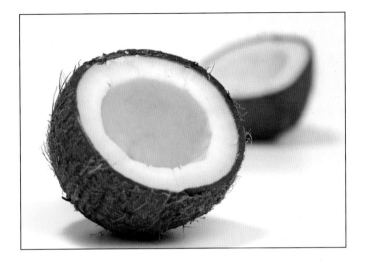

Tree of Life' since practically all of its parts can be used to support life. It's rich in fibre, and vitamins, and minerals, has been used for many things such as cups, decorative ornaments, buttons, and the fibre of the husk, called coir used to make ropes, mats and brushes. Many children happily make music with coconut shell halves, and radio programmes create the sound of horses' hooves with these. At home we have a coconut shell bird-feeder in our garden.

It's light and fibrous husk allowed the coconut to drift to other parts of the world where it could propagate. In India, where it's also known as 'The Tree of Life' priests give out coconuts to women who wish to fall pregnant.

Over the years the coconut has been recognised not only for its nutritional benefits but also its health benefits. Coconut oil was, and still is, used widely in Asian and Pacific traditional medicine. In fact, it is known as a cure-all by Pacific Islanders.

Coconut oil remedies

- **Sore skin** – Coconut oil has long been used to ease sore skin from sunburn, dermatitis, or pimples. It can help to heal skin and treat skin infections. For this reason it's commonly found in commercial skin products. Apply coconut oil to the affected area as required. Turmeric, which is anti-inflammatory, can be mixed with the coconut oil if desired
- **Dandruff** – Many cases of dandruff are caused by a fungal infection and coconut oil is thought to have anti-fungal properties. Massage coconut oil into the scalp, and leave overnight. The following morning rinse hair. Repeat this nightly as required or do each night to keep dandruff at bay
- **Premenstrual syndrome (PMS)** – Some women find that taking one to two teaspoons of coconut oil on the day when PMS symptoms usually occur helps to relieve and prevent symptoms

- **Dry skin** – Possibly the most well known use of coconut oil. Apply twice a day to treat dry skin, leave for ten minutes before rinsing off in a shower. Apply daily to maintain soft and supple skin. Massaged into the feet relieves dry skin, and tired or sore feet
- **Scars** – Coconut oil rubbed into scars, for example following surgery, for three to four minutes a few times a day can help these heal more quickly and lessen scarring. Some people find that coconut oil reduces the appearance of stretch marks
- **Warts / verrucas** – Rub coconut oil directly onto the wart or verruca, and repeat this each day until cleared. Alternatively, apply coconut oil to the pad of a sticking plaster, place this over the wart or verruca and leave overnight

Fighting athlete's foot

Coconut oil can help to treat athlete's foot. It's thought that caprylic acid in the oil has anti-fungal properties. Simply apply coconut oil to the affected area twice a day, and leave until dry.

Conclusion

In Sanskrit the name for the coconut palm is 'kalpa vriksha', translated this means 'the tree which provides of the necessities of life'. This is so true. From the coconut comes food providing good nutrition and health benefits. It also provides something to eat food from, and with, and raw materials to make other useful implements. It's a good source of fuel too.

Coconut oil, as you've seen, can be used to treat so many common minor ailments, quickly and effectively. Moreover, it smells nice too, unlike some treatments. So, you may not have a lovely bunch of coconuts in your kitchen, but just make sure you have some coconut oil available.

CRANBERRY

Over recent years the humble cranberry has moved from the domain of the alternative therapy arena very much into conventional mainstream medicine. It is one food that has a growing amount of scientific research to support its health benefits. This is something to be celebrated, and appropriate as traditionally it's at times of celebration that cranberry makes an appearance. Despite all the talk about cranberry, it may come as a surprise to learn how it may help with more than just cystitis.

About cranberries

The process of growing to collection of cranberries is impressive. Grown on low vines in peat bogs or marshes that have been drained of water, these are covered with a layer of sand since a chance discovery identified that cranberries grow larger and juicier when sand blew over them. Harvesting is in autumn and there are two methods – dry and wet. With dry

*"Only the best
make it"*

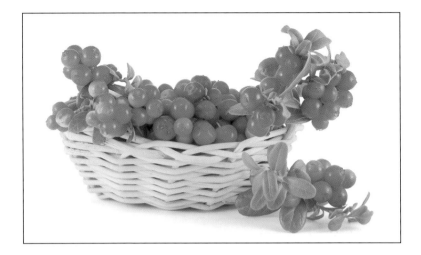

harvesting a machine that looks somewhat like a large lawnmower combs the berries from the vine and transports them along a conveyor belt to a collection bag. Wet harvesting is more efficient, and more dramatic. The bogs are flooded and a machine known as a 'giant egg beater' churns the water dislodging the berries, which float to the surface – the image of this was recreated at Kew Gardens by covering the large lake with cranberries, it was a most impressive and astonishing sight. The berries are then corralled using large wooden booms and sucked by a machine off the water into trucks. Some cranberries are harvested a few weeks earlier, when they are still white in colour, and then used to make white cranberry products.

Cranberries are a source of vitamin C, fibre, and manganese, and a very rich source of antioxidants. Their powerful antioxidant benefits are thought to be helpful regarding keeping the heart and circulation healthy, in addition research suggests that they can raise levels of good cholesterol in the blood. Research continues into their heart health benefits, and also into a possible immune-boosting and anti-cancer role too.

But it's their role in fighting infection that has really been interesting. Research suggests that by stopping bacteria sticking cystitis, gum disease, and stomach ulcers may be prevented.

Did you know?

Whether or not a cranberry is deemed suitable for a future in foods or juice doesn't just depend upon its appearance. It has to be a good bouncer too. An early New Jersey cranberry grower, John 'Peg-Leg' Webb, first noted this quality of cranberries. His wooden leg prevented him from carrying his cranberries down from the barn loft so he poured them down the steps. He found that only the best made it down to the bottom. This lead to the development of the cranberry bounce separator that's still used

today to identify the best cranberries. To pass the test each
cranberry must bounce seven times over four-inch
wooden barriers.

Cranberry history

The Delaware Indians in New Jersey revered the cranberry as a symbol of peace. Indeed, when the Pilgrim Fathers arrived the Native Indians, who are believed to be the first people to use cranberries as food, shared their knowledge of how to live off indigenous plants. In celebration of surviving their first winter the Pilgrim Fathers and the North American Indians feasted on turkey and cranberries and other foods, the first Thanksgiving celebration in 1621. They also used cranberries mashed together with deer meat to make a survival cake, called pemmican, which could be kept for long periods of time.

Cranberry and its juice even then had a role in health being used to bathe wounds and in a poultice to draw out infection from wounds. Just as the British sailors would eat limes to ward off scurvy, American sailors would eat cranberries. The juice was also used as a natural dye for blankets and clothes.

Known as Sassamanash by the North American Indians, the Pilgrim Fathers gave cranberry its modern name. To them it looked like the head of a crane bird, and so it became the crane-berry, and later the name we know it by today.

During the last century cranberries found their way into many commercial food products, the first ready-to-serve sauce being introduced by Ocean Spray in 1912. Since that time cranberry has become a familiar sight at family gatherings, and more recently as a wide range of juice beverages in refrigerators around the world.

Cranberry remedies

- **Mouthwash** – Using a commercial or home-made juice rinse the mouth for thirty seconds
- **Boils** – Make a poultice of cranberries by stewing these until soft. Apply to the affected area for ten to twenty minutes. Repeat two to three times a day as needed. Whisky can be added and some believe this makes it more effective
- **Corns / calluses** – Mash one or two handfuls of fresh cranberries and using a bandage secure these over the corn or callus. Leave for twenty to thirty minutes. Repeat daily as required
- **Haemorrhoids** – Cranberries can be used to ease uncomfortable haemorrhoids, commonly known as piles. Blend a cup of cranberries then wrap a tablespoonful in muslin and place against the haemorrhoids for thirty minutes. Repeat as necessary. Some suggest inserting the muslin containing cranberries into the rectum for an hour, removing and replacing with a new one for a further hour. If doing this be sure to leave enough of the material to get hold of so it can be safely removed

- **Dry chapped lips** – Cranberries can help to ease the discomfort of chapped lips. Take a dozen cranberries and microwave these for a couple of minutes. Mash these, allow to cool, strain, and store in a jar or other suitable container. Apply to the chapped lips. A teaspoon of honey and/or a teaspoon of almond oil may be added to the cranberries before microwaving if desired
- **Freckle remover** – Place crushed fresh cranberries onto the freckles for ten to twenty minutes and then rinse the skin with plain water

Fighting cystitis

Over the past ten years or so research has identified the potential benefits of cranberries in treating, and preventing, cystitis. It's down to compounds called proanthocyanidins, thankfully also known as PACs. These bind to the bacteria preventing them from attaching to the bladder. Consequently the bacteria are then literally, flushed away. Research suggests drinking 250mls of cranberry juice in the morning, and another of the same in the evening will provide the benefits.

Conclusion

The cranberry has literally come a long way by the time it reaches our kitchen, or our table. When I think about the times I've sat around the table with my family celebrating Christmas, or nowadays any time when turkey or even chicken are on the menu, the cranberry sauce or jelly has been somewhat in the background, with other foods taking centre stage.

It may be a small berry, but it's packed with goodness and so very versatile. Might I dare to liken it to a reserved philanthropist? It offers and gives so much, but quietly without any fanfare. Well I'd like to sing its praises and say a cranberry should not just be for high-times and celebration days, it should be for everyday.

CUCUMBER

Who doesn't immediately think of crust-less sandwiches or hidden eyes when cucumbers are raised in conversation? I know I do. The image of well-to-do ladies sipping tea from china cups accompanied by a plate of cucumber sandwiches, or reclined wearing a slice of cucumber over each eye is relaxing in itself. So long as there's one in your kitchen, you can enjoy the benefits too and remain as cool as a cucumber.

About Cucumber

Most of us think of cucumber as a vegetable but in fact it's a member of the gourd family along with squash and watermelons, and is actually classified as a fruit, scientifically known

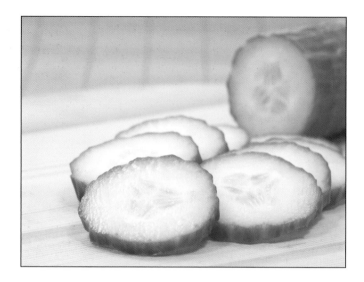

as *Cucumis sativus*. Cucumbers that are eaten fresh are known as slicing cucumbers, often found in sandwiches or salads. It's also included in a number of cooked dishes, or pickled as the smaller cultured varieties that include gherkins.

Cucumber is a rich source of water and fibre and also contains health beneficial vitamins A, B6, C, K and folate, and nutrients including potassium, iron, manganese, magnesium, and tryptophan which is converted in the body into the mood lifting hormone serotonin. A firm smooth cucumber also makes an adequate rolling pin!

Did you know?

Eating cucumber can help reduce high blood pressure that contributes to heart attacks and strokes. Cucumbers are a good source of potassium and it's this that has been found to help lower blood pressure. Cucumber skin is a rich source of fibre that can help lower cholesterol too, which in turn helps keep the circulation healthy.

Cucumber also helps people lose weight since it's low in calories and can be very satisfying.

Cucumber history

Cucumber has a long history of being used to treat skin complaints. This was made popular in Ancient Egypt, Greece, and Rome. The Romans used cucumbers to treat bad eyesight – similar to their common use today for treating sore and tired eyes. They also used cucumbers to treat scorpion bites, something most of us are unlikely to encounter.

The cucumber itself didn't find its way to Europe until the Middle Ages. It was popular for women wishing to fall pregnant to hang a cucumber around the waist. Once the cucumber had done the job and her child was born the cucumber would be discarded.

It is reported that Columbus first introduced cucumbers to the New World during his travels and that cucumbers were introduced into the United States by settlers in the 1600s. In England it wasn't until the Nineteenth Century that cucumbers were first cultivated in greenhouses. Of course, today they are produced in many countries around the world, notably China which is the biggest producer.

Cucumber remedies

- **Soothe tired and sore eyes** – Probably the most well-known cucumber remedy used for many years. Puffiness around the eyes and eye soreness can quickly be relieved by placing a chilled slice of cucumber over the closed eyelids. The cooling effect reduces swelling and it's thought that vitamin C and caffeic acid in cucumber help reduce swelling and prevent water retention
- **Skin toning** – When your skin is feeling a little under the weather cucumber can help to give it some tone. Dice a cucumber and puree it. Drain the juice through cheesecloth into a clean container and add a couple of teaspoons of honey to the cucumber juice and store in the refrigerator. Apply the mixture with cotton wool to the skin of the face, leave to dry
- **Sunburn and skin irritation** – Vitamin C and caffeic acid in cucumber help reduce swelling and ease irritation caused by sunburn, dermatitis, and other irritating skin conditions. Place a slice of cucumber against the sore skin or grind cucumber into a paste and then apply to sore area of skin. Repeat this as necessary. Eating cucumber also helps by providing liquid that hydrates the skin
- **Constipation** – Cucumbers are a rich source of liquid and some fibre, and have a mild laxative effect that helps overcome sluggish bowels. Consume one quarter of a medium sized cucumber and repeat daily as required
- **Fluid retention** – As a diuretic cucumber helps to remove excess fluid from the body and can help cleanse the bladder
- **Hair restoring** – Cucumber can provide nourishment to lank hair. Mix together one half of a peeled small cucumber with one egg and four tablespoons of olive oil. Apply the mixture to the hair and leave for ten to fifteen minutes before rinsing out. Done monthly this can help improve the texture of hair
- **Cooling** – On hot days eating chilled cucumber provides a cooling effect on the body and also provides often much needed fluid

Fighting pimples

Amongst the many benefits cucumbers bring to the skin is getting rid of unwanted and unsightly pimples. Grate some cucumber and apply to the skin. Leave for about twenty minutes and then gently wash it off the skin.

Conclusion

This wonderfully shaped fruit can be enjoyed in so many ways. A natural cleanser it brings benefits to the body both inside and out. Popular for treating skin complaints and improving the appearance of skin and hair, it's a simple ingredient for dishes and remedies.

The cucumber is one of my all-time favourite fruits as I love its crisp and crunchy coolness when eaten straight from the fridge or in a sandwich. What's more to benefit from its healing properties you don't have to be well heeled yourself.

Epsom salts

I think it's fair to say that most people have heard of Epsom salts. My relatives and friends have often referred to 'a dose of salts' when in need of relief from one ailment or another. It's interesting to note that this salt serves two distinct but related purposes. For humans it is recognised as a very effective laxative. For plants it is used as an effective fertiliser. Isn't it wonderful how Mother Nature provides?

About Epsom salt

For me Epsom salts is, in entertainment terms, the 'producer' ensuring that everything runs smoothly and goes to plan with a great end product. For years it's been used as a constituent of bath salts where it helps relieve tired and aching muscles, and of course, feet. It's also well known for its laxative effects and around the world it is used for this purpose.

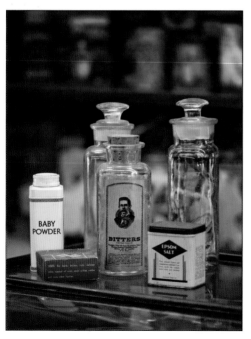

Epsom salts are principally made up of magnesium and sulphate, and it's in the hydrated form of magnesium sulphate that these are known as Epsom salts.

Magnesium performs many roles within the human body. It is involved in regulating the function of numerous enzymes, and is also necessary for normal muscle and nerve function. Magnesium also aids the use of calcium within the body and can help lower blood pressure, in turn helping to lessen the risk of heart attacks and strokes. Magnesium sulphate is used to treat eclampsia in pregnant women to lessen the risk of seizures and maternal death. However, it is important to note that it is magnesium sulphate that has been shown in research to offer these benefits, and not Epsom salts.

In the garden magnesium sulphate also

has important and productive roles. Magnesium is involved in the making of chlorophyll, helps a plant absorb phosphorus and nitrogen, and is needed for seed germination. The sulphur component may help enhance the effectiveness of plant nutrients and may also assist in the production of chlorophyll. Magnesium sulphate also helps to correct any deficiency in the soil. Gardeners will confirm how when fertilised with Epsom salts flowers such as roses bloom more and pepper plants grow larger.

Did you know?
Epsom salt can help to keep bathroom tiles free of dirt by simply mixing half a teaspoon of Epsom salts with washing-up liquid and using this mixture to clean the tiles. Epsom salts also acts as a barrier to slugs when sprinkled around those plants that are a focus of a slug's unwanted attention, helping to keep these away from plants. It also helps to keep grass lawns green.

Epsom salts history

No prizes I'm afraid for guessing that the name Epsom salts originates from the town of Epsom in Surrey. Around the time of Shakespeare it was noted that boiling mineral waters from a saline spring in the historical spa town gave rise to Epsom salts, even though the use of the salt goes back to Greek and Roman times.

Although now manufactured in many parts of the world Epsom salts retains the name of which we are all familiar. Moreover, to this day Epsom salts is used to bring relief from many different health complaints.

Epsom salts remedies

- **Sore muscles** – Whether these are bruised or strained soaking them in Epsom salts can help to relieve the discomfort. Add a few tablespoons of Epsom salts to warm bath water and relax. Alternatively, make a paste of Epsom salt with hot water and apply to the affected area. Leave for ten to fifteen minutes and then wash off well
- **Constipation** – Probably the most well-known Epsom salt remedy is for relieving constipation. It's best to follow the dosage directions on the packet, but if this is not possible dissolving a teaspoon of Epsom salt in a cup of warm water and then drinking it should do the trick
- **Skin exfoliant** – Epsom salt can be used directly onto the skin to exfoliate and then washed off. Alternatively mix a pinch of Epsom salt with olive oil and rub onto the skin, washing off after exfoliating
- **Foot odour** – This can be relieved with an Epsom salt foot bath. Add one or two tablespoons of Epsom salt to a bowl of warm water and then allow the feet to soak for ten to

fifteen minutes. Doing this also softens rough skin and soothes tired feet, and may help to treat fungal toenail infections too

- **Splinters** – To help draw out a splinter soak the affected area in Epsom salt
- **Hair conditioner** – Mix together half a teaspoon of Epsom salt with hair conditioner then apply to scalp and hair. Leave for ten to fifteen minutes and rinse out thoroughly

---

Fighting blackheads

Despite their name these are not caused by dirt, but by the build up of dead skin cells and sebum. Add one teaspoon of Epsom salts to hot water, allow to cool to a temperature that can be tolerated by the skin, and apply to the blackhead using a cotton bud. Leave for five minutes and then rinse thoroughly. This helps to loosen and subsequently remove the blackhead.

Conclusion

What a useful member of the household Epsom salts is for treating minor health ailments. A sprinkle onto the skin, into bath water, or into the intestine sorts out all manner of problems. Whether it's the body or the garden being on the receiving end, when Epsom salts are around you're practically guaranteed of more productive results.

Fortunately, it's no longer necessary to live in or near Epsom itself to gain the benefits, but it is necessary to have some to hand when needed. So don't be without it in your home.

FEVERFEW

Feverfew does what it says on the label and makes fever less. Obvious really, isn't it? Not rocket science but science is something that this simple herb does have behind it, which is why there's much more to its name than first meets the eye. In fact, this helpful herb has a number of benefits when looking to keep ailments at bay.

About feverfew

Having gone through a time of being in the shadows feverfew is now powerfully back on the scene. Scientific research has strongly suggested that this herb can help to prevent migraine headache when other, often conventional treatments, do not succeed. Although these claims are far from being carved in stone many believe these benefits to be down to active chemicals found in its leaves. One of these, called parthenolide, is able to prevent fluctuations in levels of the hormone serotonin, fluctuations that are involved in the spasm and relaxation of blood vessels that in turn result in headache. Parthenolide also affects the activity of other chemicals involved in headaches, and indeed those involved in inflammation, helping to

"A remedy for so many"

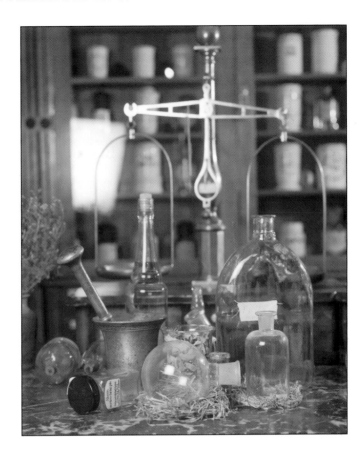

explain why it can help to relieve arthritis pain and painful periods. In fact, there are many other chemicals found in feverfew that have anti-inflammatory effects.

Feverfew has practical uses too. Although an attractive plant, and a member of the daisy family that's often confused with camomile, its strong and bitter smell is disliked by insects, including bees. For this reason, feverfew is often found in gardens performing the role of insect repellent, whilst providing aesthetic enhancement. This strong and lasting odour is used to freshen the air and when its blossom is made into a tincture this can be used both as an insect repellent but also as a natural balm to relieve itching and discomfort should insects manage to creep through these defences and bite.

Did you know?
It's Mrs A Jenkins, the wife of a retired Welsh doctor, who is credited with discovering the use of feverfew as a migraine remedy having heard about this from a local coal miner.

Feverfew history

Feverfew has gone in and out of favour over the years. Popular in Ancient Greek times the Greek physician Dioscorides is said to have recommended its use, one use being to aid menstruation and relieve accompanying unpleasant symptoms. Today it is still used by some women for this purpose, and in Mexico the plant is used in sitz baths to ease menstrual discomfort and cramps. In Ancient Greek times it was also given during childbirth to assist in the expulsion of the placenta. Another use was to treat melancholy, which in those times is believed to have included disorders such as headaches.

The name feverfew comes from the Latin 'febrifugia' which means to 'drive out fevers'. So, it comes as no surprise to learn one use is just 'what it says on the tin'.

Feverfew has always been used to reduce high temperatures and treat fever, and although with the availability of modern drugs it may no longer be the most effective, some still use it for this purpose.

After the Seventeenth Century the herb went out of fashion, hardly being used at all during the Eighteenth and Nineteenth Centuries, but towards the end of the Twentieth Century, with scientific research in the 1980s shouting about its potential to prevent migraine headaches almost overnight a renewed interest in feverfew was born.

Feverfew remedies

- **Minor skin irritation** – The anti-inflammatory effects of feverfew can be put to good use to relieve minor skin irritations such as itching. Make an infusion of dried leaves, and allow this to cool. Then apply to the affected area as a compress
- **Sore joints** – A compress of feverfew leaves can be beneficial in relieving sore and swollen joints. Soak a clean cloth in a freshly brewed infusion and apply to the affected joint. The compress can be held in place for twenty to thirty minutes with a bandage if desired. When more than one joint is affected it may be simpler to consume a cup of weak feverfew tea
- **Fever** – Long used to reduce fever it is thought that this effect is mediated through the action of compounds in the herb that prevent the release of fever-causing chemicals within the body
- **Colicky abdominal pain** – Applying a poultice of the herb cooked in a little oil to the affected area of the abdomen can help relieve abdominal discomfort
- **Painful periods** – The anti-inflammatory and blood flow promoting effects of feverfew can be used to ease painful periods. It is suggested to drink a weak infusion of feverfew on the days leading up to a period and on the days of the period
- **Anxiety** – Since feverfew has a mild sedative effect it can be used to relieve anxiety and stress. Some people use it overcome tension headaches, as it not only reduces the stress causing the headache but also helps relieve the headache itself

Fighting headaches

Feverfew is most well known for the prevention of migraine headaches, but can also be used to relieve the headache pain and nausea when these occur. Many people suggest chewing two or three leaves each day to prevent migraine headaches, others suggest that chewing one leaf each day is sufficient. However, the leaves have an unpleasant taste so often it's easier to make an infusion of the dried leaves and drink this, or to eat the leaves in a sandwich. Another reason for choosing these alternatives is that chewing these leaves can cause mouth ulcers over time.

Conclusion

It's always reassuring for me when a herb that traditionally has been used to treat health complaints is confirmed in scientific research to actually do the job. Particularly when that condition causes many people a great deal of pain and misery, and can be a difficult condition for even conventional medicine to get on top of, such as is often the case with migraine.

Nowadays, of course commercial feverfew remedies are available too for those wanting a little more convenience, but this shouldn't mean there's no benefit in having feverfew available around the home, ready to use when ailments come your way. After all, how often have you gone to the medicine cabinet and found that you're out of painkillers.

FIGS

The preserver of modesty is how I like to think about this simple fruit. Yes, its leaves are made reference to regarding this, but in health terms it can also be pretty embarrassing to be struggling on the toilet and figs can certainly be of help with this predicament. But figs have so much more to offer than assisting the call of Mother Nature. Considered a modest fruit, their fanfare should really be trumpeted.

About figs

It's true to say that mention figs and the first response is likely to be a smile and some toilet humour. After all, they do stimulate the bowels and indeed, they do this very effectively, something that was recognised long ago by the Prophet Muhammad who made mention of figs helping to prevent haemorrhoids, which as I'm sure you are aware, are often caused by constipation.

Like many people my memories of figs are of these odd looking fruits making an annual appearance at Christmastime. If figs did appear at other times of the year my impression was this would be within the realms of the truly health conscious individual, the person for whom

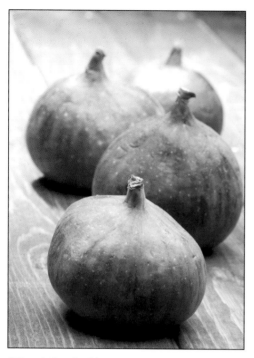

"Never judge a book by its cover"

muesli was a staple, before becoming trendy. Now figs have come into the limelight, their well publicised and tremendous health benefits having launched them into a position where they are a more regular household member, if you'll excuse the pun.

Figs are a member of the mulberry family and although there are at least eight hundred types of fig the one that most people are familiar with is the common fig, botanically called *F. Carica*. In addition to being a very tasty fruit to eat alone or with other fruits and cereals, figs are commonly used to sweeten dishes, and I'm rather fond of fig jam.

Figs have great nutritional value, one of the reasons why they've become so popular. In addition to their rich fibre content that helps the bowels to function well, they are a very rich source of calcium and of disease-fighting antioxidants. Figs are also a source of copper, manganese and potassium.

Did you know?

It's thought that fig leaves seen in paintings and sculptures of nude figures were added years after these works of art were completed by collectors and exhibitors in order to prevent any embarrassment of those viewing.

Fig history

Figs are one of the oldest fruits know to man with their remnants having been found in excavation sites dating them to as far back as 5000BC. The Romans were great fans of the fig and encouraged cultivation of new types. Figs continued their journey across the world being introduced to the New World by the Spanish explorers, and by the Twentieth Century the fig industry had become a thriving one in the United States.

Of course one of the most famous references to figs is in the Bible where fig leaves are described as being used by Adam and Eve to preserve their modesty. In fact the fig tree is the first plant to be mentioned in the Bible, and some say that it may not have been an apple that was eaten by Eve and offered to Adam, but a fig itself.

This practice of preserving modesty with fig leaves has continued through the ages. Often seen in paintings and sculptures of nude figures in current times leaves, not always fig leaves, continue to be commonly used to save embarrassment and preserve modesty in adverts, and also to raise a smile in comedy sketches when the leaf will often vary in size and be prone to an autumn behaviour of slipping off.

Fig remedies

- **Boils** – Make a paste of figs and apply to the boil. This can also be used to treat minor wounds and sores. An alternative is to roast a fresh fig, then half it. Place the soft inner part against the boil, and keep in place with a clean dressing. Leave for a couple of hours. Do this twice a day making use of one half of the roasted fig each time
- **Warts** – Press half a freshly sliced fig against the wart and fix in place overnight. The fig can also be mashed so it becomes mushy and applied to the wart
- **Facial booster** – Take the flesh of one fresh fig and mash together with full cream. Continue adding cream and a little fresh water to achieve the consistency of a lotion. Wash the face with plain water and dry. Then apply the mixture of figs and cream evenly onto the facial skin and leave for five to ten minutes. Rinse off with plain cold water
- **Arthritis** – A fig poultice can bring relief to sore muscles and joints. Soak four figs in water and then mash these into a poultice. Apply directly to the affected area and keep in place with a clean cloth or dressing. Leave for thirty minutes to an hour, and repeat this as needed

Sagging facial skin

Sagging facial skin can be problematic and is more likely to occur as we get older. It's also likely when we are feeling tired and run-down because of trying to burn the candle at both ends or because of illness. For a simple facial pick-me-up puree three to four figs and add half a dozen drops of freshly squeezed lemon or orange juice. Apply to the face and leave for around twenty to thirty minutes. Rinse gently with cold water.

Conclusion

So there you have it. It may not be the prettiest fruit when dried but it is a little dynamite, packed with goodness. Figs themselves help to preserve our modesty in so many ways by keeping the bowels moving freely and easily, by being full of health maintaining nutrients, and by being so versatile when it comes to helping to alleviate minor ailments.

In days gone by the phrase 'not give a fig' became a popular way of expressing a lack of care or concern for something or someone, and is still used today. I'd suggest that we should give a fig because much as in the past this simple fruit may have not been considered worth a great deal by some, it's clear that the truth is quite the contrary.

So, to coin and adapt another well-known phrase remember that a fig is not just for Christmas, it's for life.

FROZEN FOODS

Very few people nowadays will not have some frozen vegetables in a freezer. Usually found amongst other frozen foods such as ready meals and ice cream, frozen vegetables are as comfortable in the freezer as ice cubes. Always ready to use frozen foods are convenient, and not just for eating either.

About frozen peas

Frozen peas are possibly the most common frozen vegetable to be found in the household freezer. Even though other vegetables are readily available in frozen form – spinach, carrots, and sweetcorn, for example – if you were to go and look in your freezer right now I'd expect a bag of frozen peas to be present.

Let's not forget frozen fruits too – blackberries, blackcurrants, raspberries – are just some of the fruits I recall my family freezing, in addition to vegetables, when harvests from our allotment had been bountiful and we'd given away as much as we could.

It's not only the fact that they are there when you need them, and are a tasty food of course. Frozen vegetables in general have a long shelf-life adding to the convenience they offer. Freezing is a safe way of preserving food since at these low temperatures any pathogens present are inactivated.

When inflammation is causing swelling and discomfort something cold applied to the affected area helps to calm things down and bring relief. In fact, the 'RICE' technique is

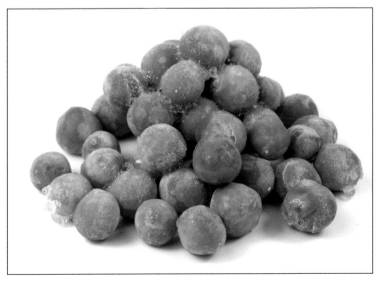

"Never be without these"

advised where 'R' is for rest, 'I' is for ice, 'C' is for compression, and 'E' is for elevation. A bag of ice cubes wrapped in a cloth and applied to the affected part works very well. But sometimes frozen vegetables are better because they're already in a convenient pack and mould to the shape of the affected part. This is why I think frozen peas or frozen sweetcorn is ideal. At least, a mixed bag of these two vegetables was just the job when I stepped out of my back door and twisted my ankle. This simple bag of frozen vegetables had a most calming effect on the swelling appearing around my ankle, and it has to be said, on the language coming from my mouth.

Did you know?
When people used to put steak on a black eye the benefits came from the meat being cold rather than meat itself. Cold helps to keep swelling down and by constricting blood vessels decreases the bleeding under the skin that causes a bruise.

Frozen food history

Long before modern refrigeration techniques became available food would be stored in cold stores in order to preserve it. Where possible food would be stored in ice, and still to this day in some Arctic communities food is preserved in holes dug into the ice.

Commercially food has been frozen since the early twentieth century, initially using the cold-pack method. In this method food was packed in large containers and these placed in cold storage rooms until frozen. However, the slow process of freezing in this way allowed water in the food to crystallise into ice, which in turn resulted in damage to the food and a loss of some of the food's taste when thawed.

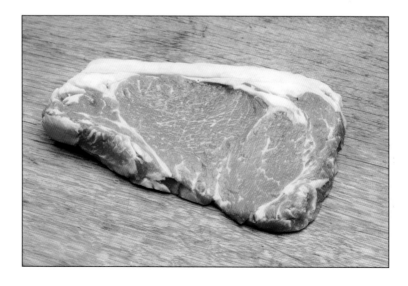

"Best eaten"

It is Clarence Birdseye who is considered to be the man responsible for modern freezing techniques. He invented the process of quick freezing, which enabled food to retain its flavour once thawed. This process was taken up by the General Foods Corporation in the late 1920s and the rest, as you say, is history. Nowadays the food industry uses 'flash-freezing' to freeze foods very quickly.

Frozen vegetable remedies

- **Breast tenderness** – This commonly occurs before and during a period, or when breastfeeding. Wrapping a bag of frozen vegetables in a soft cloth, such as a tea towel and placing this against the breast for five to ten minutes helps to relieve discomfort
- **Headache** – A bag of frozen vegetables wrapped in a soft cloth and placed against the scalp where the headache is felt is soothing. It may be easier to rest the head on the frozen vegetables by lying on these
- **Piles** – Despite popular myth sitting on a cold surface does not cause piles. However, sitting on a bag of cloth-wrapped frozen vegetables for about five minutes can help relieve any discomfort caused by piles
- **Sore joints** – The swollen painful joints caused by the many different types of arthritis, for example gout, osteoarthritis, and rheumatoid arthritis, can be eased with the cold therapy provided by a bag of frozen vegetables wrapped in a cloth
- **Nosebleed** – Cold helps to constrict blood vessels and so stop bleeding. Once again, wrapping a bag of frozen vegetables in a soft cloth, and applying to the bridge of the nose helps stop a nosebleed

Fighting ankle sprains

A simple, practical, and inexpensive approach to easing the pain and relieving the swelling of an ankle sprain is a bag of ice or frozen vegetables wrapped in a cloth and placed over the painful area. Frozen peas or sweetcorn are good because these mould to the shape of the ankle. A cold bottle of drink placed against the ankle can also help, and is probably more likely to be available to you when playing sport, until you have a cold pack to use. You can also soak a clean cloth in cold water to make a cold compress and use this. Add a few drops of witch hazel or arnica to this to help treat the bruising.

Conclusion

It's all about convenience really. This is what frozen foods bring to our lives. The convenience of having 'fresh' vegetables readily available, the guarantee of good flavour, and of course, an instant remedy for a range of common ailments.

Essentially what you've got in your freezer is something cold to calm down the most inflamed situation. This may be the fact that guests have turned up unannounced and need feeding, or something was forgotten during the weekly shop, or as is often the case in the rush of modern day living something has got twisted and needs instant relief.

Even if you're a fresh vegetable person, who dislikes the idea of frozen, do have at least one pack of frozen vegetables, or fruit, in your freezer because when you need it, it's best to be prepared.

GARLIC

Garlic is a wonderful ingredient but mention garlic and negative connotations often spring to mind. The sinister image of Christopher Lee as the vampire in Hammer's legendary movies being kept at bay by a string of garlic. Garlic and its pungent odour, a tool for keeping away unwelcome amorous advances, is often seen in comedy sketches. But there's a lot of good to be had for our health from garlic, often called 'Nature's aspirin'.

About garlic

Garlic is a member of the onion family, being closely related to the onion, leek, and shallot. The bulb is made up of individual cloves and has a spicy and pungent flavour used for seasoning. Fresh garlic is generally odour-free but when chopped or crushed or chewed a chemical reaction is triggered that converts alliin within garlic, into allicin, a sulphur-bearing compound that's responsible for its familiar taste and odour. Allicin is believed to be responsible for the medicinal benefits of garlic.

Some scientific studies have demonstrated how garlic supplements can lower blood cholesterol levels, whilst others have shown garlic supplements not to be of any benefit in achieving this. So with regards cholesterol lowering, it is currently unclear how beneficial garlic may be. There's also no conclusion over garlic's ability to help lower blood pressure either as studies have been inconsistent. Saying this, it's unlikely to do any harm so many people think it worth having plenty of garlic in their diet.

Recent research claims to have cracked how garlic may help to keep the heart healthy suggesting that when allicin reacts with red blood cells, hydrogen sulphide is produced. Hydrogen sulphide (responsible for the smell of foul eggs and used to make stink bombs) relaxes the blood vessels, which in turn reduces blood pressure, reduces pressure on the heart, and allows oxygen-carrying blood to flow more freely. Since high blood pressure is a major risk factor for heart attacks and strokes, it becomes a little clearer just how garlic may help.

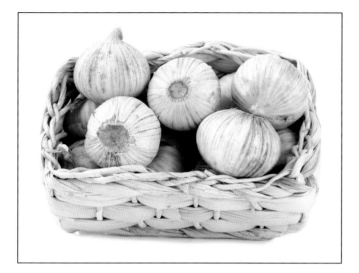

"A natural healthy flavouring"

Did you know?
When cooking with garlic, cut the cloves finely and leave for around ten minutes to enable the allicin, the important chemical for health, to develop before adding garlic to recipes.

Garlic history

Garlic has a long history of medicinal use. Garlic remedies were used in India five thousand years ago and Chinese medicine has acknowledged garlic's therapeutic value for thousands of years.

Egyptian pyramid builders were paid in fresh garlic, to maintain their strength and stamina, and it's said to have been chewed by Greek Olympian athletes – suggesting how its now perceived benefit in supporting a healthy circulation may have been recognised in those distant times. Roman soldiers inserted cloves of garlic between their toes to prevent athlete's foot on long marches.

With regards the powerful effect of garlic in treating infection as recently as 1858, Louis Pasteur recognised the antibacterial powers of garlic, and during the First World War, doctors used garlic juice to prevent wounds becoming septic.

Garlic remedies

- **Coughs and colds** – Garlic has antiviral properties helping to fight coughs and colds. Add some grated fresh garlic to warm water and drink. Honey and lemon can be added too if desired
- **Wound infections** – Its antibacterial effects help to heal wound infections. There is

also some scientific evidence to suggest that garlic may help in the seemingly never-ending battle against the hospital super-bug MRSA

- **Athlete's foot** – Garlic has been used to treat fungal skin infections such as athlete's foot for many years, a usage dating back to at least Roman times
- **Heart attacks** – May keep the heart and circulation healthy. This is vitally important because, in the UK alone, about a quarter of a million people suffer a heart attack and about 145,000 people suffer a stroke every year
- **Strokes** – It is thought that the allicin from garlic may help lower blood pressure, lower cholesterol levels, and reduce the chance of blood clots. Because of this, garlic help lessen the risk of someone suffering a heart attack or stroke

Fighting colds

Garlic is probably most renowned for its potential to stave off viral coughs and colds. One study has demonstrated that taking a supplement of garlic each day lessened the chance of suffering a cough or cold by more than half. Moreover, those taking garlic who still succumbed to a cold made a speedier recovery and were less likely to suffer subsequent cough and cold infections.

Conclusion

Generally speaking, one or two cloves a day are believed to provide health benefits. To help stem a cough or cold, around three cloves a day is often recommended. Overall, it remains unclear whether garlic can actually lessen the risk of someone having or dying from a heart attack or stroke but garlic is felt to be safe and many believe it's worth considering, either as a supplement or in its natural form. As a seasoning, it's certainly healthier than salt, which is known to raise blood pressure.

HORSERADISH

Yorkshire puddings and roast beef are what jump into my mind when horseradish is mentioned because that's how I was first introduced to this sauce, and that's still how I most enjoy its unique flavour. With that said, I'm partial to a dollop of horseradish in a cold beef sandwich too. These days I can enjoy more of it, something I struggled to do when much younger when I also hadn't learned how it can be a useful treatment for minor ailments.

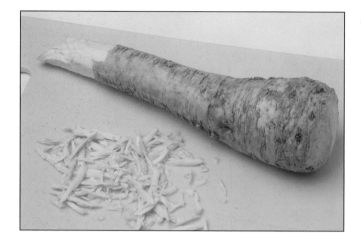

"Beef's best friend"

About horseradish

I love the anticipation of the biting flavour horseradish brings, not only to myself, but to others sitting around the meal table. I remember Sunday lunches with my family watching to see whose eyes would start to water first, the indicator that they had perhaps overdone it with the horseradish.

Responsible for the pungent taste of horseradish, and so its sometimes entertaining effects, is a compound called allyl isothiocyanate. This is produced by involving another compound, called sinigrin, in a chemical reaction, which is initiated when horseradish is chewed and mixed with liquid such as saliva. So now you know why your eyes water and your nose runs when you eat horseradish, and indeed other members of the *Brassicaceae* family, such as mustard and wasabi, something else I've recently been introduced to and enjoy.

It's no surprise to me that I've always enjoyed the eye-watering taste of horseradish so much. Growing up my mum always put a little mustard in ham sandwiches, but wondered why the mustard pot emptied so quickly. The reason was my brother and I would challenge each other with how much mustard we could tolerate in these sandwiches.

But it's not only its taste that's good about horseradish. Nutritionally it's beneficial too being a source of potassium, calcium, magnesium, and vitamin C. Moreover, one tablespoonful of horseradish has just six calories and no fat and as such in the United States is recommended as a part of a healthy low-fat diet. In fact, synthetic allyl isothiocyanate is used as a topical anaesthetic, and has antibacterial properties, which helps to explain some of its benefits when treating minor ailments.

Did you know?
In Japan horseradish is known as 'western wasabi', and is often dyed green and substituted for the more expensive wasabi.

Horseradish history

Horseradish has been used for treating health complaints for centuries. The Greeks used it as a therapeutic rub for lower back pain, and also as an aphrodisiac. For some time it was considered a cure-all; being used as a cough expectorant, as a soothing remedy for irritated skin, and of course, as we know too well, to relieve sinus congestion. In fact, it's reported that in more recent times its health benefits were exploited by those of the American South who are said to have rubbed horseradish on the forehead to relieve headaches. Some compounds in horseradish also have antibacterial properties, which helps explain how horseradish may help treat boils and other skin infections.

It wasn't until around 1640 that horseradish was eaten by the English, seen as a food for the less wealthy classes, such as labourers. It was grown and served to travellers as a cordial at inns and coach stations to combat exhaustion and provide them with renewed energy for their next journey. However, by the end of the Seventeenth Century all were eating it, as an accompaniment to beef, and in fact oysters too.

I've often wondered how horseradish got its name. One source suggests it began life as a 'sea radish' because in German it's called 'meerrettich' and the English mistakenly pronounced this 'mareraddish'. Subsequently it became what we all now know and love, horseradish. Another source suggests it was originally known as 'redcole' in England, and 'stingnose' in some parts of the United States, a name that describes its effects well.

Although the white-creamy beige colour sauce made from grated horseradish root and cream is familiar to most of us as a popular condiment, particularly in the United States, it was only as recently as 1860 when sales of bottled horseradish began. But now its growing popularity means it's common throughout the world where it's used not only as a condiment but also forms an important ingredient in other foods, for example in soups.

Horseradish remedies

- **Acne / Boils** – Horseradish can help to calm down inflammation and treat minor skin infections. Add two tablespoons of grated horseradish to half a cup of honey and leave overnight. Apply the mixture three to four times a day with cotton wool to the affected skin until healed
- **Arthritis** – Horseradish is thought to work by irritating the skin which then encourages blood flow to relieve inflammation. Boil a cup of milk and mix in two tablespoons of grated horseradish. Soak a clean cloth in the mixture and apply to the affected area. The mixture when cooled to a tolerable temperature can also be massaged into the sore joint or muscle
- **Aching feet** – Take one or two horseradish leaves and gently blanch these. Remove any fibres running through the leaves and then strap to the bottom of the feet with a bandage. Leave for around thirty minutes. This may also help treat fungal foot infections
- **Headaches** – To one tablespoon of finely grated horseradish add half to one

tablespoon of water. Wrap in a muslin cloth and apply to the area of the headache. Some say that sniffing freshly grated horseradish can also help relieve a headache

- **Itchy skin** – Horseradish juice can help to relieve irritated and flaky skin. Juice slices of horseradish and add to honey – how much depends upon the area of skin affected. Apply to the affected areas
- **Toothache** – Grate horseradish and apply to the gums near to the aching tooth
- **Stings** – Apply a slice of horseradish root to the sting for around twenty to thirty minutes followed by ice for a further five to ten minutes

---

Fighting congestion
Horseradish has been used for centuries to relieve nasal congestion and as an expectorant for clearing mucus from the chest. Slicing horseradish root and breathing in deeply may achieve the desired effect. Chewing slices of horseradish in the mouth usually promotes relief of congestion. Begin with a small slice and increase the amount as needed.

Conclusion

I suppose it shouldn't come as a surprise to learn that a food with such concentrated and powerful effects upon the body can be harnessed to provide healing benefits for minor health complaints. Such a convenient food it is too.

Much as I've enjoyed horseradish sauce for many years I have to hold up my hands and say I hadn't realised how helpful horseradish could be for treating minor ailments until researching this book. It really is a very useful food to have available and if I needed an excuse to have more of it around, I'm pretty sure I now have it.

ICE

The clink of ice in a glass, the deep sigh of relief from a painful joint, this solid water is a wonderful substance that we perhaps take for granted but throughout time has served us well. It's helped keep food in a state where it can still be enjoyed, keeps drinks refreshingly cool, and can really be of benefit in a crisis, whether that be a physical crisis when we've put a foot wrong, or a social one where without ice available we are likely to, metaphorically speaking.

About ice

On a hot summer's day ice is welcome as we enjoy the coolness it brings to drinks. Often at weddings and parties ice sculptures will take centre stage – I remember being amazed and full of sympathy when in blistering hot weather I watched ice sculptors in Thailand creating

"Cools the most heated situations"

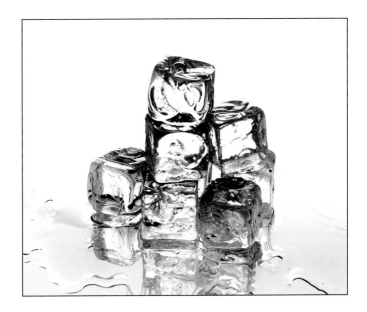

the most magnificent winged bird out of ice, racing to finish before Mother Nature inter-fered. Not so long ago I had the pleasure of visiting Norway where the most amazing icicles were there for all to see. Ice also provides the basis for many sporting activities, for example, ice skating and ice hockey. On the other hand, however, during winter ice may not be as welcome as it slips us onto our bottom with a thump.

Around the home ice plays an important role too, even if ice is no longer necessary in most homes to preserve food as refrigeration has taken over this role. However, whilst staying with friends recently I was reminded how having ice available is helpful when accidents occur. My friend's black Labrador likes to dig shallow holes in the garden, in the lawn to be precise. The fact that my friend's lawn is a rolling lawn, and the holes are small, means they're not easily seen. You've probably guessed what happened. An agonising scream drew my atten-tion to the fact that my friend had twisted her ankle having inadvertently stepped into the hole. I knew how painful this could be having done something similar whilst stepping out of our backdoor some years back. It was frozen vegetables that saved the day for me then, and ice that saved the day for my friend, who fortunately had an ice pack in the freezer just for this sort of occasion, which I was to learn later, had happened once or twice before. So ice is a cool healer.

Did you know?
A paper cup of water kept frozen in the freezer until needed can be used to relieve a painful swollen joint. Peel away the paper and massage the ice against the affected area. As the ice melts away peel back more of the paper cup and continue massaging.

Ice history

Over the years probably the most important role for ice was as a method of keeping food produce cool. There is reference as far back as 1100BC to the Chinese using ice houses, and the Greeks and the Romans also made use of the benefits for food preservation.

In more recent times ice would be harvested and then delivered door to door for home-owners to use to prolong the survival of food. Early refrigerators were known as ice boxes because they contained a block of ice, something that was still used in the 1940s. In fact, many people still call portable coolers that accompany picnic outings or visits to the beach 'ice boxes'.

As commercial refrigerators became available the role for ice changed from being a purely functional one of keeping food fresh, to a more social one of being added to drinks to keep them cool or used in the preparation of food stuffs such as smoothies.

Nowadays refrigerators are a common part of many people's lives, and many refrigerators now have their own ice-makers incorporated in them. However, it's still common to see bags of ice for sale since when having a party ice is one of the essentials added to cool and freshen drinks, added to an ice bucket to maintain wine at an appropriate temperature, or placed in a cooler to keep drinks cold whilst outdoors or away from home.

Ice remedies

- **Sunburn** – Uncomfortable sunburn can be calmed by applying ice wrapped in cloth to the affected area. The ice lessens the blood flow to the affected area, reduces swelling, and numbs the area a little too
- **Cold sores** – Many people report that ice can help to stop a cold sore in its tracks. Apply an ice cube to the area where the cold sore appears as soon as the tell tale tingling starts
- **Toothache** – Sucking and rolling an ice cube around the mouth can help to relieve uncomfortable toothache
- **Shaving nicks** – Applying an ice cube to a bleeding shaving nick can stop the bleeding by constricting the blood vessels, slowing the blood flow, and allowing a clot to form
- **Headaches** – Wrap some ice in a clean cloth and apply to the area affected by the headache
- **Hiccups** – Sipping ice cold water or eating ice cubes are two remedies that have been used for many years to relieve hiccups. Some suggest rubbing the ice cube on the outside of the neck over the throat
- **Haemorrhoids** – The pain and discomfort, and itching, caused by haemorrhoids can be relieved by sitting on a bag of ice wrapped in a clean cloth. Despite popular myth, sitting on cold things doesn't cause or make haemorrhoids worse

Fighting sprains

A sprain is an injury to a ligament, a common example being an ankle sprain – a strain on the other hand is an injury to a muscle or tendon. Often sprains cannot be avoided but they can be easily treated using the 'RICE' technique – Rest, Ice, Compression, Elevation. Ice decreases blood flow to the area, relieves swelling, and lessens inflammation. This is where a bag of ice, or an ice pack, comes in very handy indeed. Sometimes a bag of ice cubes – place a dozen cubes in a zip-lock bag – is better because this can mould to the shape of the affected part of the body. Whichever is used, wrap it in a clean cloth and apply to the injured part. You can massage the area with ice directly but keep the ice moving, never leave ice directly against the skin or there's a risk of frostbite.

Conclusion

So there you have it, ice really is cool. It should always be available in your refrigerator for when you need it. Unexpected guests may need a cooling and refreshing drink, or there may be something to celebrate requiring an ice bucket to keep the bubbly chilled. The celebration in question may simply be the arrival of summer and its hot days. Or as is often the case ice may be needed to calm down an inflamed joint, or an inflamed situation.

Such a simple part of nature ice has fulfilled its changing role admirably throughout the centuries. No doubt it will continue to do so in the future, provided we let it, because climate change is having a huge impact on the ice we all know and love.

LAVENDER

Lavender has become a very important flower for me. I've recently introduced it into my front garden where its rich lilac colouring, unique scent, and rather gangly appearance always leaves me feeling happy when I set off for work and return home again. This alone should make it an essential in my opinion, but there's more, so much more to lavender than first meets the eye, or, more often than not, the nose.

About lavender

Lavender has had a chequered history with me. Even though it's one of the most calming herbs this hasn't always been its effect on me in my life. As a child it's the scent I remember wrapping around me as I walked up my grandmother's driveway, and as my visits to her were always very good my earliest memory of this herb is a happy one. But time moved on and like most teenagers I wanted to assert my independence so finding a lavender bag hanging on a coat-hanger in my bedroom clothes cupboard did not please, or relax me. Now

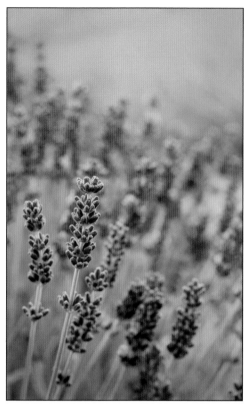

"Welcome home"

that I have lavender in my front garden greeting me each day and instantly bringing back the happy memories it's a favourite again. It goes without saying that I don't have it in my cupboards.

I think my experiences are similar to those of others when it comes to lavender. After all, lavender is used in a host of products – fragrances, soaps, bags, and cushions, some of which can be heated and used to relieve aches and pains. So it's unusual not to have something of lavender around the home, whether this is in a bag or tied in bunches and hung upside down.

Bees make a high quality honey from lavender and sugar, sweets, and ice cream, amongst other foods are flavoured with lavender. Chefs use lavender as an ingredient in a number of foods and dishes, particularly in France, and enjoy making good use of lavender's sweet flavour that comes from the flower buds – it's in these that the essential oil of lavender is found providing its familiar scent and flavour.

Did you know?
Lavender bags are not only effective at turning a musty smelling cupboard into a sweet smelling one. They are also effective at repelling moths.

Lavender history

For thousands of years the scent from the essential oil of lavender has been utilised to soothe and relax the mind and spirit, to calm nervousness and excitability. Simply smelling the scent is often enough. Inhaling the aroma from a lavender infusion is another way of reaping the benefits. Physical symptoms such as rapid breathing, heart palpitations, muscle tension, headaches and stomach butterflies, when related to anxiety, can be brought under control and calmed with lavender.

Ancient Greeks called lavender 'nardus', after the Syrian city of Naarda, and this herb has long held a reputation as a holy herb being used in the preparation of holy essences. Lavender's position of respect was also reflected in its value. In Roman times the cost of lavender flowers were said to be the equivalent of fifty haircuts from the local barber. A tradition that existed in Roman times and still is popular today is to add lavender to baths to facilitate a relaxing experience.

There's even more to lavender than just a sweet and soothing scent. It doesn't just calm down an emotionally inflamed mind. It can also calm down physical inflammation too. This is put to good use when treating minor skin ailments such as minor burns, insect bites, and dermatitis. And if that isn't enough, lavender is antiseptic. During the Great War (World War 1) lavender was used for this purpose to disinfect floors and other surfaces in hospitals. More recently in hospital some research has found that receiving inhaled lavender in oxygen after having an operation can improve pain control post-operatively.

Lavender remedies

- **Stress** – Probably the most well known use for lavender, relieving stress. Smelling fresh lavender in a garden or packing a pillow with lavender can help calm the mind and body. Commonly used lavender essential oil can be added to a pillow, pyjamas, or a handkerchief for daytime use. Inhaling the steam from a hot lavender infusion, drinking this, or adding lavender to a warm bath and soaking in this can all help ease stress
- **Abdominal problems** – Nausea, indigestion, and wind can all be eased by drinking a cup of lavender tea
- **Minor cuts and wounds** – Lavender is a good antiseptic. After making a lavender infusion using the flowers, strain and leave until the temperature is at a level tolerable to the skin. Apply directly to the affected area or as a compress
- **Sore muscles** – Lavender has good anti-inflammatory effects and an infusion can be used to soothe tired and aching muscles and joints. Make a compress and apply to the affected areas. Lavender infusion can be rubbed into the affected area to stimulate the circulation, which in turn helps to relieve inflammation
- **Headaches** – Lavender can help to relieve headaches, particularly tension and stress-related ones. Make a lavender infusion and inhale the steam. Drinking the lavender tea can also help
- **Skin complaints** – The anti-inflammatory and antiseptic properties of lavender can help to heal minor sores, and other skin complaints such as dermatitis

Fighting insomnia

Insomnia is a problem for many people, with difficulty getting off to sleep a common complaint. Lavender filled pillows have long been used to relax the mind and body, moving these to a state where sleep can come more easily. Some scientific evidence now supports the effect of lavender in slowing down the nervous system, promoting relaxation and refreshing sleep. It can also help to lift mood.
An alternative to a lavender filled pillow is a relaxing lavender

infusion consumed around thirty minutes before bedtime. Infuse three lavender flower heads in boiling water for three to five minutes and then when at a tolerable temperature drink.

Conclusion

It's been a little windy today whilst I've been writing this chapter. Not digestively I hasten to add, although lavender would have probably dealt with that. No, the weather has been the stimulus for my lavender to be gaily dancing in the breeze. Their tall gangly appearance swaying to and fro makes me think of fashionable teenagers at a pop music festival, crammed together, moving to the beat, and relaxed and content. Yes, that's what lavender does for most of us, and I like my teenager analogy, I think it works. Provided that is, that when these teenagers get home again, someone hasn't hung a bunch of lavender in with their clothes.

LEMON BALM

I have always loved lemons. For as long as I can remember I've reached into my emptied glass for the slice of lemon and chewed it eagerly. Its sharp taste is something that many can't tolerate, and my behaviour often attracts gasps of surprise, but not disgust, I hope. But I enjoy the saliva releasing anticipation, the self-challenging bite, and then the freshness it leaves in the mouth. But you don't have to run the fresh lemon gauntlet to gain benefit. Lemon balm can bring similar rewards in perhaps a more leisurely, and soothing, fashion.

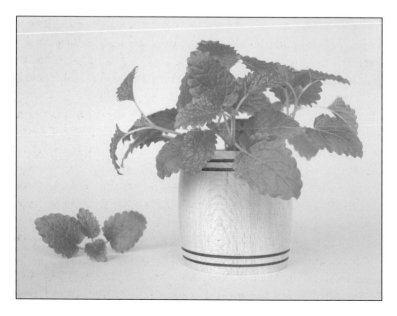

"A refreshing way to lift the body and mind"

About lemon balm

What a wonderful lemon aroma is perfumed through the air by the leaves of lemon balm. Rub these leaves and the scent becomes stronger. Chew the leaves and the mouth is filled with a wonderful lemony flavour, making it useful for freshening the mouth and helping to battle bad breath. The volatile oils in lemon balm relax the mind and body, specifically the muscles, and can help to lift mood when feeling a little low. Rubbing crushed lemon balm leaves onto the skin acts as an effective insect repellent too.

A member of the mint family lemon balm is also known by its botanical name *Melissa officinalis* and also as Melissa herb. The word 'Melissa' means 'honey bee' in Greek and its little white flowers are very attractive to bees that are able to produce good honey from it.

Lemon balm can often be found in foods such as ice cream and sweets where it's used as flavouring. It may also be used to garnish salads and other dishes. As a herbal tea is how most people recognise it, and indeed may have used it. More recently, its effectiveness as an antiviral treatment for treating and preventing recurrences of cold sores has been used such that it now appears in commercial treatments for this purpose.

Did you know?
Ancient bee keepers would rub crushed lemon balm leaves on their beehives to encourage bees to return to the hives and bring other bees along too.

Lemon balm history

The lemony scent is refreshing, but also soothing, a benefit put to great use in calming and lifting the mind. It has long been used to help relieve anxiety and ease depression related to childbirth and the menopause. Dioscorides and Pliny recognised and made use of its medicinal healing and relaxing properties. Since ancient times it was believed to completely revive a person, particularly from those complaints resulting from disorders of the nervous system, including those known today as being of the mind.

The Romans were kind enough to bring it to Britain, amongst their many other great ideas. Quickly it appeared to gain a reputation for being able to treat practically all health complaints. Said to renew youth, improve brain function – memory in particular – and chase away melancholy and sadness, and even cure baldness, those of years gone by may well have been right. Research over recent years has suggested that lemon balm can boost memory, helping those who consumed lemon balm each day to learn, store, and retrieve information reinforcing something that was postulated a few hundred years ago. And if you've ever smelled the lemon scent – and like it of course – then you're bound to have felt a little happier, possibly even merry and joyful as lemon balm was described as leaving people.

Today many still swear by its ability to promote longevity. In the Seventeenth Century Carmelite nuns in Paris created Carmelite water, a distillation of lemon balm leaves, including lemon peel, nutmeg and angelica root, which was used as a perfume. In recent years a number of people who have lived well-beyond one hundred years attribute their longevity to consuming Carmelite water, known originally as 'aqua mirabilis', or miracle water.

Lemon balm remedies

- **Depression** – Lemon balm has long been used to lift someone out of depression, whatever the cause of this might be. Drinking a warm lemon balm herbal tea a couple of times a day can help
- **Indigestion** – Some people suffer indigestion when they are feeling anxious or stressed. Lemon balm herbal tea can relieve these symptoms, and relax a person, helping to eliminate not just the symptoms but the cause of the indigestion, that is, the stress. This can also help those suffering with stress-related irritable bowel symptoms
- **Bad breath** – Drinking lemon balm herbal tea can help freshen the breath directly and indirectly by reducing stress, which makes bad breath worse. Sometimes iced lemon balm herbal tea is more effective
- **Swollen joints** – Soak a clean dressing in an infusion of lemon balm and apply to the affected joint as a warm, or cold, compress as desired
- **Skin sores** – Lemon balm can help to soothe minor skin lesions when applied as a cream. Chop up a few leaves and mix with yogurt until this has reached the consistency of a cream. Apply to the affected area. Storing in the fridge can help as this provides an additional cooling effect on the skin when used. Alternatively, after soaking a lemon balm herbal tea bag in hot water for three to five minutes once it has reached a tolerable temperature apply it to the affected area
- **Chest congestion** – Lemon balm herbal tea can help reduce mucus production and ease irritating catarrh

Fighting cold sores

Lemon balm has effective antiviral properties, thought to be due to the polyphenols found within it. It has been found to be particularly useful in the treatment and prevention of cold sores. Scientific research using lemon balm has demonstrated a decrease in the duration of a cold sore attack, and a reduction in the frequency of attacks. Lemon balm is thought to prevent the herpes virus getting into the cells.

After allowing a lemon balm herbal teabag to cool this can be applied to the sore. Alternatively lemon balm can be applied as a cream.

Conclusion

I always find it fascinating, and to be perfectly honest reassuring too, when something that has been used historically and anecdotally has shown itself to be of benefit, begins to be confirmed by modern science.

Such a simple herb, lemon balm is often thought of as a humble plant, despite its rich and powerful scent, and medical benefits. I still vividly remember learning that there was something effective to offer those with uncomfortable, and for many soul-destroying, cold sores and the delighted look on the face of one of my patients when I was able to pass this information on. The benefits of lemon balm stretch further than just the lips, so be sure to have some within reach.

LEMON JUICE

Lemons are full of zing and provide a wonderfully refreshing drink, not forgetting they're an excellent source of vitamin C. Who amongst us doesn't reach for lemon juice when we are suffering with a cold or cold infection. However, the benefits lemons bring go far, which is why whether it's to sprinkle over pancakes or to soothe a sore throat having lemons in the kitchen is essential, particularly if you don't want to be left feeling a bit of a 'lemon'.

About lemons

There's something about lemons that just makes you feel happy. The fact that they conjure up images of calm and tranquillity is a little odd since the bitter taste of lemon can sometimes cause a sharp intake of breath. But the fact is talk about lemons and summertime, cool lemonade, and for me, the beach, is what comes to mind. Another reason why lemons make me smile is that growing up my brother and I would use plastic Jif lemon containers, once

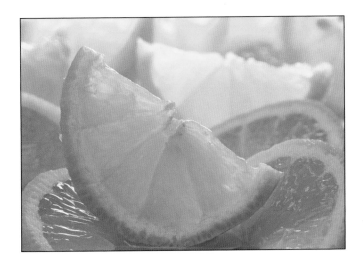

"Adding zest to life"

the original lemon contents were used up, to squirt each other with water. A family friend of ours called these the pacifist's water pistol!

When cooking lemon adds a tangy flavour to many dishes, including soups and salads, and cakes. Fresh lemon is often squeezed onto fish once served – always squeeze lemon gently to begin with to confirm the juice is heading in the right direction.

Citrus limon is the scientific name for this fruit that is a rich source of vitamin C, important for a strong immune system, wound healing, and for helping to absorb iron into the body. Vitamin C is a powerful antioxidant helping to mop up free radicals that left can cause damage to arteries and joints, and increase the likelihood of cancer developing. Lemons also contain other powerful antioxidants, flavonoids, that are recognised as helping protect the heart and circulation, and also may help protect against cancers. Other chemicals found in lemons are limonoids, responsible for the scent of fresh lemon peel and being noted in research to have potentially great health benefits. One limonoid in lemon, called limonon, has been found in laboratory studies to help fight a number of different cancers, including mouth, skin, and breast cancer by preventing cancer cells from proliferating. Limonin may also help to lower harmful levels of cholesterol.

Did you know?
Lemon juice can help to determine whether a person is an introvert or an extrovert. Scientists believe that the activity of a part of the brain that produces saliva in response to food stimulus can determine introverts, who produce a large amount of saliva when tasting lemon juice, and extroverts, who produce much less saliva.

Lemon history

Lemons were developed originally as a cross between the citron and the lime and are thought to have originated in India or China. They found their way to Europe thanks to Arabs, who in the Eleventh Century brought them to Spain, and the Crusaders who brought them to other European countries. Christopher Columbus was responsible for introducing lemons to the Americas during his many travels and voyages.

The Romans used lemon as an antidote to poisons, and ladies of Louis XIV's court kept their lips seductively red by biting lemons. In years gone by lemon juice was even used as a contraceptive.

The fact that lemons are rich in vitamin C has been used for centuries to ward off scurvy, notably amongst the sailors exploring and discovering new lands, but also amongst developers and miners during the Californian Gold Rush. Nowadays they still remain an important food not only for their flavouring in cooking but for the health benefits vitamin C provides.

Lemon remedies

- **Sore throat** – Lemon helps to clear mucus and vitamin C helps the immune system fight infection. Mix one tablespoon of lemon juice in a cup of hot water. Allow this to cool. Gargle the liquid and then swallow. Repeat this until the cup is empty. Honey can be added to sweeten and it also coats and soothes the throat
- **Skin irritation** – Cut a lemon in half and rub the flesh of the lemon against the irritated part
- **Dandruff** – Into two cups of water mix the juice of half a lemon. Apply the juice from the other half of the lemon to the hair. Wash hair with shampoo first, then rinse with water, and then with the lemon and water mixture already prepared. Repeat this daily until dandruff has cleared. In fact, a few drops of lemon juice run through the hair can provide a clean without the need for water
- **Stopping minor bleeding** – Lemon juice can curtail minor bleeding, for example, soak cotton wool in lemon juice and put into nostril to stop a nosebleed. Squeezing lemon juice directly onto a minor cut will sting, but will also disinfect and stop the bleeding
- **Boils** – Heat up a lemon in the oven or hot water, cut in half and strap half to the boil. Add one to two tablespoons of lemon juice to boiling water, allow to cool, then use the lemon and water mixture to cleanse boil and then apply a sterile dressing. Repeat daily until healed
- **Toothache** – Lemon juice applied to the painful area is soothing and brushing teeth each day with lemon juice or rubbing teeth daily with the white of lemon peel helps to keep teeth white
- **Combat stress** – sit back and slowly sip a delicious glass of lemonade. Alternatively, place slices of fresh lemon in a hand towel soaked in warm water. Roll it up and warm in the microwave. Then put it loosely around the neck
- **Sore feet** – Massage feet with lemon juice after soaking feet in hot water for ten to fifteen minutes. Rinse feet with cool water. For corns place a slice of lemon over the corn and keep it in place with tape and leave overnight. Repeat this daily until corn has gone. The same treatment can be used to treat warts too

Fighting blemishes

Applying lemon juice to a skin blemish can get rid of it. Left on overnight lemon juice is said to help clear blackheads, in fact, the juice is also used by some to rid their skin of freckles, age-spots, and wrinkles. The pulp left after juicing a lemon is also good for skin, helping to soothe insect stings and bites. Around the home, mixed with bicarbonate of soda, lemon juice helps remove blemishes from plastic too.

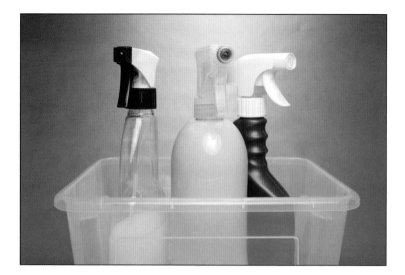

"You don't always need these to clean around the home"

Conclusion

The number of uses for lemon is extensive, both when cooking and for treating minor ailments that are likely to trouble us all at some point in our lives. Their bright yellow skin is a natural mood lifter, and the inside and outside of a lemon brings a refreshing zing to life.

Let me leave you with some of the lesser known lemon remedies that you may wish to give a try. Rubbing lemon on feet soaked in warm water may help to prevent nightmares, and rubbing lemon juice on nails and cuticles helps keep these strong. If you're feeling a little queasy scratch and sniff a lemon rind to relieve nausea, and if you think you may have had one too many drinks, be sure to rub a lemon under your armpit before falling into bed because, yes you've guessed it, some say that this prevents a hangover the following day!

LIQUORICE

Talk to people about liquorice and in my experience it's something you either like or dislike. There doesn't appear to be much grey in the discussion. But liquorice is in so many different foods and beverages, even those who don't like it as a sweet, may be surprised to learn that they are benefitting from its sweetness in other ways. Moreover, it's well established as a healer, so should really be hailed as such.

About liquorice

It's in sweets that liquorice is probably best recognised but it's involvement in foods goes much further than the pick 'n' mix sweet displays. As flavouring liquorice is widely used in Chinese cuisine, in soups, for example. Liquorice is also used to flavour some soft drinks, notably root beer, which although most common in the United States has made a welcome appearance – as far as I'm concerned – here in the UK. It's also used in herbal teas where it

"Liquorice plays all sorts of roles in our lives"

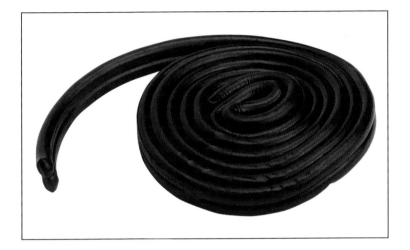

can provide a countering sweet taste to the sometimes bitter aftertaste that herbal teas bring. And whilst on the subject of drinks, in Calabria a popular liqueur is made from liquorice extract.

The liquorice plant, botanically called *Glycyrrhiza glabra*, is actually a legume being related to peas and beans. The name it's known as in the UK, liquorice, comes from the Ancient Greek words meaning 'sweet root', which of course it is, and often chewed as a sweet itself. Liquorice root is used as powder and also made into teas and tonics. The extract of liquorice is obtained by boiling its root and allowing most of the water to evaporate.

For a long time it's been used as an ingredient in medicines, once again to exploit its sweet flavour in disguising the sometimes unpleasant taste of a medicine. Mary Poppins sang, 'just a spoonful of sugar', but she'd have been as wise to sing just a mouthful of liquorice.

Did you know?
The active part of liquorice root is glycyrrhizin which is responsible for its sweetness. In fact, glycyrrhizin is around fifty times as sweet as the sugar sucrose.

Liquorice history

Liquorice appears to have always been a popular food and ingredient in drinks. Large amounts were discovered in Emperor King Tut's tomb confirming that it was popular with pharaohs, whilst its appearance within Egyptian hieroglyphics confirms it was popular amongst those of lesser standing too. Caesar and Alexander the Great are said to have hailed the wonders of liquorice, and soldiers used it whilst marching.

In traditional Chinese medicine liquorice has been used for centuries for the treatment of respiratory complaints such as laryngitis, bronchitis and asthma. It is thought to have anti-inflammatory and anti-allergy properties making it useful for treating these health conditions. Today it is a very popular component of Chinese treatments, with some sources suggesting it is second only to ginseng in its frequency of use. Even in Western medicine liquorice finds a role where it is often found in cough remedies and used in medicines to disguise unpleasant flavours. A substance in liquorice called licorione is thought to lower stomach acidity and lessen the amount of stomach acid secreted.

Until recently once extraction had taken place the waste root was disposed since it was thought to have no further use. However, it is now being used in the manufacture of chemical wood pulp, which in turn can be pressed into boards and used to make boxes.

Liquorice remedies

- **Mouth freshener** – Chewing on liquorice root helps to freshen the breath and overcome bad breath
- **Indigestion** – It's the flavonoids in the liquorice root that are believed to be responsible for its soothing effects on the lining of the stomach helping to relieve indigestion, and heal stomach ulcers. Taking powdered liquorice in water can help to relieve attacks of indigestion and liquorice root can also be boiled in hot water to make tea.
- **Dermatitis** – Liquorice has been used successfully to treat dermatitis and minor skin infections when used in a poultice and applied to the affected area
- **Mouth ulcers** – These are often painful making eating food and drinking liquid difficult. Sucking on liquorice and rolling the liquorice around the mouth ulcer can help relieve the pain as liquorice has anti-inflammatory effects
- **Constipation** – Liquorice is a mild laxative and can be used to ease the passage of bowel motions when these have become a little sluggish. Chew and swallow liquorice or mix half a teaspoon of liquorice root powder with warm water and drink. Liquorice tea can also be used
- **Gut spasm** – This often occurs in irritable bowel syndrome and when a person is suffering with anxiety. Liquorice has an antispasmodic effect on the gut so when chewed and swallowed, or taken as powdered root with warm water, or as warm tea made from liquorice root, can help relieve uncomfortable bowel spasm. It can also help to relieve bloating and wind
- **Premenstrual syndrome** – Menstrual cramps can be eased by taking powdered liquorice root in warm water, as it is believed to have mild oestrogenic effects

Fighting coughs and sore throats
Glycyrrhizin within liquorice has anti-inflammatory properties that help relieve a sore throat and irritating cough. It is said to be as effective as the drug codeine as a cough suppressant, but without the possible side effects associated with codeine. Rhizomes in liquorice when mixed with water soothe an irritated throat. It is

also an effective expectorant helping to clear mucus from the throat and lungs. Mix powdered liquorice root with warm water, then gargle, and swallow.

Conclusion

Its rich black appearance, and chewy consistency, makes liquorice a sweet that often is an acquired taste. But once acquired this taste is unique and rewarding. As we've seen it's not just its sweet flavouring that has been exploited over the years. For centuries its medicinal benefits have been recognised for easing discomfort caused by inflamed parts of the body. Its role in smoothing the passage from irritating dry cough and sore throat to resolution is still to this day being used, amongst the other health benefits it brings.

Such a simple root to have available and to use, it really should take pride of place in the kitchen. When we need it, it will help out, in all sorts of ways.

Warning:

Consuming too much liquorice may damage the liver and circulation, and may increase blood pressure and cause oedema. This is particularly the case if consuming too much concentrated liquorice sweets. It may also cause headaches and lethargy and shortness of breath.

OATMEAL

Make sure you get your oats. I'll let you decide for yourself how you wish to interpret that well-known phrase. Suffice to say, getting your oats, on a daily basis is beneficial in more ways than one. From my own experience doing this makes me feel good inside because I associate it with ski-ing, and a terrific way to get a day on the slopes off to a great start. At home my family has porridge a few times a week, and sitting down with my family always brings a smile to my face. Just thinking about it makes us feel warm inside, and it's true, oats are really good for our insides as you'll find out. And they are also very good for our outside too.

About Oatmeal

For something so small this cereal grain provides so much for so many. Food for humans, fodder and bedding for animals, and simple treatments for minor ailments. Processing of oats by rolling or crushing produces the familiar oatmeal. Although probably best known as breakfast cereals porridge and muesli, oatmeal is also used as an ingredient in a variety of cooked foods including biscuits and cakes, one of my favourites being flapjacks. Occasionally oats are used to brew beer. An acquired taste I've found.

Since oats are rich in carbohydrates they're a great provider of energy, so a bowlful first thing in the morning should keep the average person happy until lunchtime as oats cause blood sugar levels to rise slowly for a few hours providing sustained energy, and can stabilise mood too. In addition, during the process of digestion soluble fibre in oatmeal forms a gel that delays the movement of food from the stomach. This causes us to feel full longer, so we're less likely to feel hungry, and as a bonus, this can consequently help with losing weight. Eat and lose weight, sounds like the Holy Grail of health.

This gel also helps to trap cholesterol-related substances, preventing the cholesterol from being absorbed into the body. The effect of this, as science has demonstrated, is to reduce levels of harmful cholesterol, and importantly to lower levels of harmful low-density lipoprotein or 'bad' cholesterol. Moreover, oats are a good source of antioxidants, notably vitamin E, zinc, and selenium. Some research also suggests that antioxidants in oats make it less likely that fatty plaques will be formed on the artery walls. It's these plaques that are responsible for narrowing the arteries, obstructing blood flow, which results in heart attacks and strokes. So all in all research has shown that those who eat more oats are less likely to develop heart disease.

The health benefits of oats extend even further than the fact that they are a rich source of soluble fibre. They're doubly beneficial because they also contain insoluble fibre. This may help to fight cancer and, what it's most well known for, relieving constipation. It achieves this because it doesn't dissolve in water, but acts like a sponge, absorbing water, making stools larger and so speeding their passage to the outside world. With regards the gut some people with irritable bowel syndrome find that their symptoms are prevented by increasing the amount of fibre in the diet, however, others find that doing this worsens their symptoms.

Indirectly oats benefit our emotional well-being too. Let me share with you a personal example of this. For me the thought of a bowl of porridge conjures up a feeling of warmth, like sitting on a rug in front of an open fire, wearing your favourite winter sweater with your arms wrapped around your body. Feels good doesn't it?

Did you know?

Oats can help overcome sweaty feet, a complaint most of us suffer from time to time. Often it's just inconvenient, but sometimes it can be very embarrassing. It doesn't help that each foot has more than a quarter of a million sweat glands, and we tend to lock our feet up in shoes and socks day after day. Feet are one of the sweatiest parts of the body and can produce more than a pint of sweat each day. A simple remedy is to place oatmeal in the socks which will absorb excess moisture.

Oatmeal history

The history of oats is not entirely clear. It's believed that they probably originated in Asia Minor, but for a long while remained as a weed. Swiss cave findings of oats suggest they were

"Get some oats"

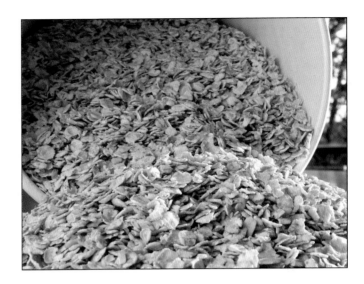

cultivated in the Bronze Age. It's said that in the time of the Ancient Greeks and the Romans oats were considered to be diseased wheat.

For many years there were differing opinions as to the value of oats. Used as fodder for horses and other animals some declared this was all the oat was fit for. In his dictionary Samuel Johnson defined oats as 'Eaten by people in Scotland, but fit only for horses in England' to which Scotsman James Boswell retorted, 'That's why England has such good horses and Scotland has such good men!'

Now, however oats have an established position in everyday diet, being accepted as offering numerous health benefits.

In 1997 the Food and Drug Administration (FDA) in the United States of America permitted those foods containing a lot of oat bran or rolled oats to carry a label claiming that when combined with a low-fat diet these may lower the risk of heart disease. Since that time scientists have suggested that a diet rich in oatmeal may also lower the risk of high blood pressure and diabetes, which in turn helps lessen the risk of heart disease, heart attacks, and stroke. Thinking about the youngsters in our society research has shown that children who eat oatmeal regularly are fifty per cent less likely to become overweight when compared with those children who did not eat oatmeal. Another good reason to begin the day with a bowl of porridge.

Oatmeal remedies

- **Corns** – Particularly unpleasant if they become painful. An oatmeal water soak can help. Add a cup of oatmeal to boiling water in a ratio of around 1:15 and continue boiling until water has reduced by around twenty-five per cent volume. Strain this and soak feet in the water once cool enough to tolerate. Remove oatmeal from the strainer and use to exfoliate the feet whilst they are soaking

- **Chapped skin** – Use oatmeal as a soap-substitute to prevent loss of the protective oils from the skin that causes the skin to dry out. After washing the skin dry it by taking a handful of dry oatmeal and rubbing on the skin. This is very good for chapped skin on the hands
- **Constipation** – A well known and effective way to relieve and prevent constipation is by eating fibre, insoluble fibre that is. A bowl of porridge or muesli each morning can help keep things regular
- **Splinters** – Mix oatmeal, banana, and a drop of water into a paste and apply it to where the splinter is. Leave for four to six hours and then the splinter should be easily removed

Fighting itchy skin

Oatmeal has been used for centuries to relieve irritated itchy skin and is now included in many commercial products for this purpose because it's a very good emollient. For itchy skin caused by eczema, psoriasis, sunburn, chickenpox or other conditions make an oatmeal paste by mixing uncooked oatmeal and water, and apply to the itchy areas either directly or by placing in muslin cloth.

Adding oatmeal to the bath provides a very soothing experience for skin. Wrap two handfuls of oatmeal in muslin, tie to make a bag and then drop this in the water. An alternative that can be used for the bath or shower is to hang the bag beneath the tap or showerhead so the water passes through the oatmeal.

In addition, for the extra benefit of using oatmeal as a soap substitute use a muslin bag of oatmeal as you would use a washcloth.

Conclusion

Surprised? I expect you are! Who'd have thought that a simple breakfast cereal could offer so many wonderful things for our health and well-being? It really is something that will look after us from first thing in the morning until last thing at night, and from childhood right through to later years.

A simple food that makes a quick energy boosting meal, and can be put to good use in treating minor ailments we may be faced with. It may well make good horses, and can certainly make us healthy men and women.

ONIONS

Mention onions and the first thing that comes to mind are sore, streaming eyes. What an unfortunate reputation for the onion to be saddled with because it's a wonderful food that like itself, has many layers of use. So let's peel back some of the layers and find out how helpful onions can be in everyday life.

About Onions

The reason why onions trigger rivers of tears is because slicing breaks cells causing a chemical reaction which results in the release of a gas. This combines with water in the eye to form dilute sulphuric acid, which is very irritating to the nerves in the eyes making them sting. Tears are made in an attempt to flush out this irritant.

One way to avoid this miserable experience, which spoils the pleasure of cooking with onions for many, is to chew gum at the same time as slicing the onion or to light a candle nearby. Professional chefs swear by cutting up onions under cold running water, or sprinkling white vinegar over the cutting board beforehand. Since the root of the onion has the greatest concentration of the enzymes necessary for this chemical reaction cutting it last, instead of first which many people including myself do, can help.

For me the onion conjures up an image of a man riding a bicycle, wearing a blue and white striped shirt and a beret on his head, a string of onions draped over the bicycle handlebars. 'Mais oui', the French onion-seller. Interesting it is then to learn that the French countryman who is renowned the world over for his romantic reputation may have had more than assistance with cooking in mind when with a smile on his face he provided onions. Historically onions have a reputation of being a powerful aphrodisiac, commonly used in ancient Greece for this purpose, forbidden to be eaten by Egyptian pharaohs for this reason, and traditionally offered to French newly-weds in the form of soup the day following their wedding. Perhaps that's why I enjoy French onion soup so much!

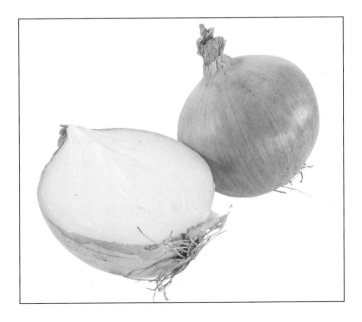

"It doesn't have to end in tears"

Onions are a rich source of quercetin, a plant pigment flavonoid. Quercetin has powerful antioxidant properties, is thought to be anti-inflammatory, and is a natural antihistamine making it very useful for treating and preventing allergy symptoms. Some research also suggests that it may also have anti-cancer effects, and that quercetin may help to relieve symptoms of anxiety and depression. Onions are a rich source of other flavonoids, of chromium, and of other nutrients including fibre, folic acid, potassium, and vitamin C, which contribute to their perceived health benefits. These include helping to protect the heart and circulation from damage by reducing levels of harmful 'bad' cholesterol and possibly by lessening the risk of blood clots forming, and also helping maintain bone strength. As a natural source of prebiotics (food needed for probiotics to thrive) they may help promote good gut and immune system function. Onions are also low in sodium and fat-free.

Did you know?
Many years ago, according to the book *1000 Places To See Before You Die* by Patricia Schultz, before it became known as the Big Apple, New York was known as the Big Onion, because it was said to be a place with many layers that could be peeled off without ever reaching the core.

Onion history

Believed to be one of the oldest known vegetables onions have been traced back to the Bronze Age (5000BC) so they really are a vegetable with a long history. Pyramid construction workers are said to have been fed onions. This may not have been only explained by the many nutritional benefits but also because Egyptian culture at that time viewed the onion with great reverence, it being seen as a symbol of eternal life. Onions were also buried with the dead, the belief being that its strong scent would bring life, more specifically breath, back.

The athletes of ancient Greece would eat large quantities of onions in the belief that doing this would lighten the balance of blood, and would rub their muscles with raw onion to firm them, something Roman soldiers are also said to have done.

Of note is that onions have been used to treat ailments for centuries. Doctors have recommended onions to help women become pregnant, one reason for this being the perceived effect on libido and in helping a man's erection, another reason might be because of the effect chromium is thought to have in balancing levels of female hormones, which is why consumption of onions may help prevent symptoms of premenstrual syndrome. Headaches – something that can also indirectly affect fertility – have also traditionally been treated with onions by placing a slice of raw onion on the back of the neck, or by boiling an onion then making it into a poultice allowing to cool before applying to the head.

Onion remedies

- **Acne / boils** – Scoop out a little flesh from half an onion cut crosswise to make an onion cup. Place the cup over the boil to help it draw. Alternatively simmer one sliced onion with honey until soft. Make into a paste, allow to cool, then apply to boil or acne spot
- **Bruises** – Place a poultice of grated onion and salt against the bruise
- **Minor burns** – Run the burn under cold water for ten minutes then cut a raw onion in half and rub against the burn
- **Sand or grit in eye** – Starting with the root of the onion cut into slices, and into small pieces. The idea is to promote tears that will naturally cleanse the eye
- **Warts** – After applying fresh lemon juice to the wart place raw chopped onion onto the wart. Leave for ten to twenty minutes. Repeat two to three times daily
- **Haemorrhoids** – Slice a raw onion and mix with one to two teaspoons of honey. Put in a fresh dressing and apply to the haemorrhoids for a few hours
- **Nausea / vomiting** – Place a slice of raw onion under each armpit

Fighting foot problems

Onions can be used to overcome a number of foot problems. To relieve tired and aching feet roasted onions mashed and applied to the feet in a poultice can help, and by including soap in this poultice corns and calluses can be also be treated. Chilblains can be helped by first soaking the feet in warm water and then rubbing the dried feet with sliced raw onion.

Conclusion

Onions, no kitchen should be without them. In fact, as a consequence of researching this chapter I'm going to grow even more myself. A nutritious vegetable that offers a distinctive flavour, many long-term health benefits, and is a pretty good first aider into the bargain.

You no longer need to be worried if the thought of onions has in the past brought tears to your eyes. Be reassured too that when it comes to romance onion breath won't be a problem if you eat some parsley. In fact, whilst we're on the subject of troublesome aromas, placing a cut onion in a freshly painted room will remove the smell of paint.

PAPAYA

Look for the bare necessities, the simple bare necessities. I can't help but think of Baloo the bear singing this to Mowgli in the Disney story *The Jungle Book* when I see a papaya. This was my introduction to the word, well, to pawpaw, which is what papaya is also known as. It wasn't my introduction to the fruit itself, however. That came much later when *The Jungle Book* was a distant childhood memory. However, both have re-emerged in my life, through my daughter. She loves the Disney story, and I'm glad to say loves papaya too. So fortunately we invariably have one or two available in our kitchen to eat, and of course that we're able to make good use of should minor ailments arise.

About papaya

The papaya is a member of the pawpaw family. Botanically speaking it's a berry, whose name is *Carica Papaya*. In fact, papaya trees are not trees at all. They are considered large herbs. Like many other fruits papaya is known by other names, including pawpaw and tree melon.

It could all become quite confusing if I'm not careful so let's get to the fleshy stuff. Papaya is a very nutritious fruit being an excellent source of vitamins A and C, and of potassium. Being low in calories, and a source of some calcium, iron, and some B vitamins, its richly coloured orange flesh makes an ideal snack, and for many is a wonderful way to start the day – which I can vouch for from personal experience.

But papaya doesn't only offer a nutritious snack or indeed, a meal itself. Papaya helps to facilitate the enjoyment of other foods too. It can do this because papaya leaves and unripe papaya contain an enzyme called papain, which is able to break down protein in meat making it more tender.

In some parts of the world it is known as the 'medicinal tree' because its seeds, that have a pepper-like flavour, have been used over the years to make medicine. Still today papaya can be used to treat a number of common minor ailments.

Did you know?
In some cultures the mature ripe papaya fruit is used as an aphrodisiac.

Papaya history

The papaya is believed to have originated in Mexico, Central America and the northern parts of South America. It is said to have been first described by Oviedo, a Spanish chronicler, in 1526. Spanish and Portuguese sailors are credited with transporting papaya seeds to other subtropical countries and hence papaya's journey began so that to this day it is grown in most countries enjoying a tropical climate.

Papain enzyme, in the unripe papaya and papaya leaves, has been used for thousands of years in South America to tenderise meat where crushed leaves would be wrapped around the meat and left overnight. Since around the 1750s the effects of the enzyme papain have been recognised. Latex from the papaya fruit is dried, and purified, enabling the enzyme to be extracted such that nowadays papain is available in many commercial meat-tenderising products found in most supermarkets.

In addition to its role as meat tenderiser papain also contributes to a number of other practical uses. It can be used in the process of shrink proofing wool, and as an ingredient in cleaning solutions for soft contact lenses. For those wanting a Hollywood smile papain is included in toothpaste as a teeth whitener. In traditional medicine it is used to assist wound healing.

Papaya remedies

- **Weeping sores** – Papaya fruit has been used for many years to speed up healing of sores. Place a slice of papaya pulp over the sore and keep this in place with a sterile bandage or sticking plaster. Change every few hours and continue until sore heals
- **Sore eyes** – Make a poultice of mashed papaya fruit and place over closed eyes. Leave for ten to fifteen minutes each time and repeat a few times a day
- **Cellulite** – Some people have found that papaya fruit can help reduce the appearance of cellulite. Mix papaya fruit with yogurt until this is the consistency of a lotion. Apply by massaging the mixture into the areas of cellulite and keep in place with cling film for twenty to thirty minutes, then remove cling film and rinse off with warm or cool water
- **Improved digestion** – The papain enzyme in papaya can help to promote good digestion and relieve and prevent constipation. Its anti-inflammatory properties also help to soothe an upset stomach. Eating the ripe fruit or making the fruit into a delicious juice are two ways of achieving these benefits. Avoid the unripe fruit as this can cause stomach upset and worsen indigestion
- **Warts** – This requires the milky latex from a green papaya to be dripped onto the wart or verruca two to three times daily until this has gone. This remedy can also be used to treat corns

Fighting skin complaints
The papain enzyme within papaya is an effective exfoliant and has also been used in medical conditions to remove damaged and dead skin from wounds, for example from burns and skin ulcers, to help speed up the healing process. It is also thought to have some antibacterial properties that help to fight infection. Applying papaya fruit directly onto the skin can act as a facial exfoliant to remove dead skin cells and as a skin cleanser leaving the skin smoother and more supple. The papaya can be applied sliced, mashed, or as a juice. Massage into the skin and allow it to dry. Leave for five to ten minutes and then rinse off gently with cool or warm water. This process can also help to reduce the appearance of age spots.

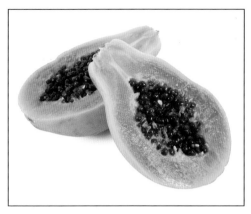

"A delicious way to put a smile on your face"

Conclusion

Papaya is a very cheerful fruit with its bright orange flesh. Cutting open the fruit reveals its black seeds that are present in abundance making this most delicious fruit a contrast of colours that shout out and immediately draw the attention.

Very few fruits, and their constituent parts, have been so researched and papain enzyme is one that as you have seen has been put to great use over recent years. This is a fruit that should be in every kitchen, and nowadays, modern cultivation and shipping means for most people this is possible. A fruit to be eaten and enjoyed and a fruit that when ailments arise can help out. As Baloo the bear quite rightly sang, look for the bare necessities, and the bare necessities of life will come to you. For me it's clear that papaya is one of these.

PEPPERMINT

Popular for flavouring gum, toothpaste, and of course, what it's most well known for, sweets, amongst a whole host of other things, peppermint is a fabulous herb to have around. It is a constituent in many over the counter remedies because it works bringing effective relief from a number of health complaints. Need I say more?

About peppermint

There's something about peppermint that I find comforting. It's not easy to put my finger on precisely what it is, but having it around is reassuring. Perhaps it's the warmth it brings internally, or the cooling effect it has when applied to the skin. It's a calmative so that may explain things or it may be simply that over the years I've realised more reasons to celebrate peppermint and so my confidence in it has grown.

This celebration and my fondness for peppermint may stem from many reasons. You won't be surprised to learn that peppermint sweets are something I'm rather partial to, a likening I've inherited from many members of my family who would always have peppermints of one sort or another with them – securely in decorated tins or free to roam inside a handbag or a pocket. In fact, it's become a habit for one of the musicians in my band to bring along a packet of mints each week when we get together and play. Moreover, I recently learned that my home is near to the oldest peppermint district in the UK so perhaps that's why I've been drawn to peppermint, quite literally.

Peppermint has antispasmodic, antiseptic, anaesthetic, and decongestant properties, so is it any wonder it is so highly respected? With my doctor's hat on – metaphorically speaking – I've always had good results with my patients who've used peppermint tea, or indeed made use of prescribed formulations of peppermint, for upset stomachs, wind, and irritable bowel syndrome.

If that isn't enough for us to be grateful for from this pretty plant – a hybrid cross between spearmint and watermint – with its purple flowers and slightly hairy stem it also produces large amounts of nectar that is utilised by honeybees to make honey.

Did you know?
It is normal for a person to pass wind up to thirty times a day.
Obviously this often goes unnoticed, thankfully.

Peppermint history

The Greeks and Romans are reported to have held peppermint in high regard. At their feasts they would adorn their tables, and indeed crown themselves, with peppermint. Their cooks would also use peppermint to flavour sauces and wines.

Peppermint is regarded by many as the world's oldest medicine. But despite being said to have been used by Greek physicians peppermint only became used in Western Europe in the Eighteenth Century. At this time its medicinal properties were quickly recognised, gaining it entry into the London Pharmacopeia in 1721.

Nowadays, of course, peppermint is one herb that few people will question is beneficial to health. This is mostly down to its rich menthol content that is effectively made use of in commercial treatments but also in home-made ones too for treating minor health complaints such as uncomfortable bloating, sore feet, blocked up noses, to name just a few of these. Menthol is believed to relax the muscles of the intestines, and dilate blood vessels in the skin.

Peppermint is also a good source of vitamins A and C, and of manganese, which also contribute to health. Moreover, science supports its use for treating symptoms of irritable bowel syndrome, helping to explain further why prescribed preparations of peppermint are available.

Peppermint remedies

- **Irritable bowel syndrome** – Whether it's bloating, excessive wind, or indigestion peppermint can help relieve these often miserable and uncomfortable symptoms when taken

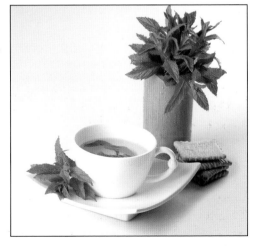

"Where ever you be, this will let your wind go free"

in capsules or peppermint tea. Peppermint can also relieve feelings of sickness and nausea

- **Congestion** – The menthol in peppermint is well recognised as helping to relieve symptoms of cold infections such as nasal congestion, as it is an effective decongestant. Menthol thins mucus and helps to break this up so that it is easier to clear from the body. It is also calming and soothing for sore throats and irritating dry coughs. Inhaling the steam of hot water with peppermint oil added is very effective, taking care not to get too close to avoid the nasal passages getting burned

- **Tired feet** – Peppermint has a cooling sensation on the skin and this is particularly beneficial for tired and aching feet. Peppermint oil can be added to natural yogurt and massaged into the feet or alternatively soak the feet for around thirty minutes in a bowl filled with warm peppermint tea, or warm water with half a dozen drops of peppermint oil added. Rubbing peppermint into the skin can relieve sore skin around the rest of the body too, not only the feet

- **Sore muscles** – Peppermint helps to soothe and relax these. Allow a cup of peppermint tea to cool and then soak a clean cloth with this. Press against the affected muscle and hold in place with a bandage

- **Headache** – Add a few drops of peppermint oil to olive oil and massage gently into the temples. Alternatively bruise fresh peppermint leaves and apply to the temples

- **Breath freshener** – Chewing fresh peppermint leaves or drinking peppermint tea helps to freshen the breath. But you possibly know this, because who hasn't disguised telltale breath aromas with peppermint sweets?

Fighting wind

Excessive wind may be funny for those who don't have it, but it's not funny if it's you who has it. Gaseous release from the human body is normal but if this gets trapped it's uncomfortable, sometimes even painful. This is where peppermint comes in very handy indeed because its antispasmodic and calmative effects relax the sphincters and intestinal muscles allowing the body to release the wind. Peppermint oil capsules (coated so they can get to the intestine and not irritate the stomach along the way) are popular, as is peppermint tea. The latter is particularly good if consumed immediately after a meal.

Conclusion

I don't mind being asked questions, but one I don't like to be asked is, 'what's your favourite. . .?' Why don't I like this question? Because I can never really decide. Generally speaking I don't tend to have a single all-time favourite of any thing, I have a number of all-time favourites. So peppermint would definitely be one of my all-time favourites, and at any one time may be at the top of the list, for example, when dealing with irritable bowel syndrome.

What's important isn't whether it's number one. What's important is that it's in the team, there to play its part which as I hope you've seen, can be a very responsible and effective one.

POTATO

Whatever you like to call a potato – spud, tattie – it's something we're all familiar with and enjoy in one way or another whether that's baked and smothered with butter or chipped and served with salt and vinegar. I doubt there's a kitchen that doesn't have a potato or two nestled in there somewhere, waiting to be eaten, or indeed, used to treat a minor ailment.

About potatoes

Potatoes are a very, how should I say, considerate food. Being rich in fibre means they assist the bowels to function properly, but are less likely to cause wind. In culinary circles they provide an excellent main course, accompaniment, or filler. Without having to think too hard it's easy to create a long list of dishes and snacks that potatoes contribute to – including some of my favourites – chips, baked, boiled, roasted, mashed, crisps, diced, in stews, pasties, shepherd's pie, and salad.

Potatoes have also been used for many years as a source of entertainment for children. I certainly remember playing with a 'spud gun', putting sticks and other objects into a potato to make potato people (commercially first sold by Hasbro as Mr Potato Head in 1952), and cutting and shaping halved potatoes to print with.

In the UK alone there are said to be around 450 different varieties of potato grown, and worldwide the number is in the thousands. Potatoes are a tremendous source of energy because they are rich in carbohydrates. They are also a good source of vitamin C, iron, folate, potassium, and vitamins B1 and B6. Moreover, despite popular misconception they are considered a low calorie food and fat-free, making them a very healthy and nutritious option.

Did you know?
Some people with Raynaud's phenomenon – a condition where changes in temperature or stress temporarily constricts small blood vessels in the extremities, for example the fingers, interrupting blood flow causing numbness, tingling, and considerable pain – benefit by having a hot baked potato wrapped in foil in their coat pocket that acts as a hand warmer, helping to lessen the risk of a change in weather triggering a painful attack of Raynaud's. When the heat has been lost from the potato it can be eaten to provide the body with energy.

Potato History

It's believed that potatoes were first cultivated by the Inca Indians in Peru around six to seven thousand years ago, who also made use of their medicinal benefits by rubbing potato onto the skin.

The English word potato comes from the Spanish word 'palata', and it was Spanish explorers who introduced them to Europe. As far as the United Kingdom and Ireland are concerned Sir Walter Raleigh is mostly credited for their introduction.

Over the years the humble potato has found favour throughout the world. In the Eighteenth Century it became popular in France during the reign of King Louis XIV, being introduced to French cuisine by Antoine Parmentier. Whilst captive in Prussia during the Seven Years' War Parmentier had little choice but to eat the potatoes offered him. Back in France he won a competition to identify vegetables that could be used to supplement those foods available during hard times. Having grown a small field of potatoes he had these watched by royal troops, as if the potatoes were a prized possession. Locals stole samples and as a result of this clever piece of marketing, potatoes became part of French cuisine, nowadays often referred to as 'a la Parmentier'.

Potatoes not only became a popular staple in the diet, for some they were very fashionable. Louis XVI of France apparently wore potato blossoms in his buttonhole as a fashion accessory.

During his presidency Thomas Jefferson served French Fries at the White House, so confirming the arrival of this particular form of potato in the United States of America.

Like many major discoveries in history the potato crisp was created by chance, actually, as a result of anger and retort. Commodore Cornelius Vanderbilt, an American railway magnate, was disgusted with the thickness of his potatoes served to him whilst dining at an upmarket restaurant in Saratoga Springs in 1853. Braver than most he sent them back to the chef. This infuriated the chef who as a retort sliced them extremely thin, fried them, and

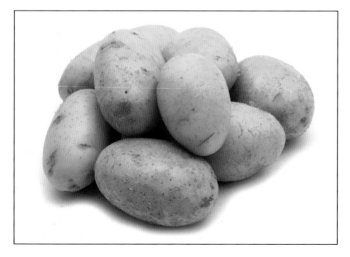

"So humble but so good for us"

covered them in salt, hoping to get his own back on the customer who'd dared to criticise his cooking. Vanderbilt delighted in his new found chips – called at the time 'Saratoga Crunch Chips' – and so potato crisps, or potato chips as they are still known in the United States, came to be.

In 1995 the potato became the first vegetable to be grown in space.

Potato remedies

- **Headaches** – Make a potato poultice by boiling one or two large unpeeled potatoes until soft, then mash. Remove excess moisture and wrap in a cloth. Then place on the back of the neck. This is also helpful for relieving discomfort of sore breasts, sore joints, and sore eyes too when placed over closed eyelids
- **Sore joints** – Potato broth can help to ease sore joints by calming down inflammation and swelling. Boil chopped up new potatoes, strain, and soak cloth in broth and apply to affected joint
- **Neuralgia** – Bake a potato, immediately wrap in a cloth to maintain its warmth, and gently place against sore area of skin. Potato can be mashed soft if desired
- **Piles and vulval varicosities** – Apply grated potato to the swollen area. Some suggest shaping a piece of raw potato into the shape of a suppository and inserting it into the rectum to treat piles but seek medical advice before trying this
- **Circles under eyes** – Extract juice from one or two potatoes. Soak cotton wool in the juice and gently hold against closed eyes for five to ten minutes
- **Skin problems** – For a scaly skin rash rub the flesh of half a potato against affected area. To ease a bruise, sunburn, or other sore skin grate a potato and apply as a poultice

Fighting warts

Potatoes have long been used to treat warts. Protagonists believe chemicals within the potato are responsible for curing warts. Slice a potato in half and rub the flesh against the wart, or cut a slice of potato and tape this against the wart overnight. Do this daily until wart disappears.

Conclusion

What a wonderful fellow the potato is to be sure. Helpful around the kitchen and around the body, and not too difficult to grow in a vegetable patch.

Like many traditional remedies handed down over the years it's difficult to pinpoint exactly why potatoes might help to heal minor complaints, and whether it's actually time rather than Mother Nature that's making the difference. However, often doing something is all that's needed to accelerate the healing process and when there's no harm in trying there's everything to gain. Moreover, with some of these remedies, as a bonus, you can actually eat what's not being used.

So, potatoes in my opinion are a very useful thing to have around, and if you'll excuse me, all this talk about potatoes has given me an appetite for a plate of fish and chips. Well, everything in moderation!

RADISH

Perfectly formed and beautifully coloured, but not always the commonest food found in the kitchen. It has a unique and quite startling flavour, is a wonderful cleanser of the palate, and has a cheerful bright red round appearance. It really is an eye-opener the radish, so it's time to open your eyes to its benefits even further.

About Radish

The type of radish that most people are familiar with is the succulent globe radish with its bright red skin and contrasting white flesh on the inside. The size of a small ball with lengthy leaves, as a child I remember these as being a good toy, when my father wasn't looking, to swing around my head and release into the air, trying hard to make this projectile fly as far as possible. Rather like the hammer throw in athletics. Anyway, enough confession from me for the time being.

Something else that I'm sure you're all too familiar with is the distinctive peppery taste. This is due to the fact that when substances in radishes are chewed and mixed with an enzyme they are converted into another substance called allyl isothiocyanate. This also gives mustard, horseradish, and wasabi their pungent flavours. This biting, and awakening flavour, is a little too powerful for some palates so people find dipping the sliced or bitten radish into salt helps counteract this. If you want to eat radishes but find it difficult to handle the flavour, try eating them early in the season when the flavour is mild, since as the season progresses so does the strength of their flavour. Alternatively, enjoy one of the other varieties such as the white icicle radish that is white and long like a carrot and milder in flavour.

Radish is usually served as part of a salad, but can also make a convenient snack in packed lunches or on picnics. It is a very nutritious food being rich in vitamin C and

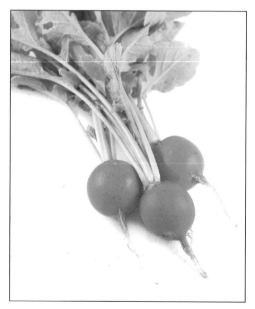

"The great cleanser"

folic acid, but low in calories. Radishes are also a good source of potassium, calcium, and some B vitamins. They can also be steamed and can be used as an ingredient in smoothies.

Did you know?

Seeds of some radishes, the oilseed radishes, are grown and then pressed to extract and produce oil. No surprise there I hear you say, the name telegraphs this fact. But hold your horses. Although this oil is not suitable for human consumption in the future it may be useful as a source of bio fuel. Now there's something to shout about.

Radish history

Radish is a member of the *Brassicaceae* family, and termed *Raphanus sativus*. The word Radish comes from 'radix', the Latin word meaning 'root'. These root vegetables originated in China thousands of years ago and then made their way to Ancient Egypt and Ancient Greece where they were cultivated. The Romans enjoyed radishes too and the journey of the radish continued such that by the 1500s they were being grown in England. It is at this time that the smaller round red radishes many of us are most familiar were first recorded. From England explorers took the radish and introduced it to North America.

Ah the great cleanser. Its fresh and pungent flavour was recognised as an effective way of cleansing the palate before a meal. The French served radishes before a meal for this purpose. Before drinking wine some people recommend eating a radish, again to cleanse the palate. In fact, one of the health uses of the radish is to overcome bad breath.

Most recently radishes in Japan made worldwide news where there was much upset caused by a daikon radish – a mild flavoured giant white radish. One was found to be growing through a pavement and receiving great admiration for this supreme feat. However, someone, or some ones, was not so in awe of it as it needed to be rushed to the intensive care unit of an agricultural research centre, the result of having been attacked by a person or persons unknown.

Radish remedies

- **Minor burns** – Mix mashed radish with crushed ice until this is of a consistency thick enough to rub over the scald or burn. After running cool water over the burn or scald apply the mixture to the affected area. Cover with a clean dressing or cling film and leave for ten to fifteen minutes. Radish juice can also be used for this complaint
- **Congestion** – The pungent flavour produced by chewing a red globe radish can help to loosen blocked nasal passages and sinuses. Repeat as needed
- **Splinter** – Tape a slice of radish to the splintered and sore area. Leave overnight and the swelling and splinter should then be gone

- **Insect bites and stings** – Cut a slice of radish and rub the white flesh against the sting to bring relief from discomfort. Radish juice can also be used for this complaint
- **Bruises** – Ideally this needs a daikon radish, but it's worth giving the well-known red globe radish a try if a daikon isn't available. Grate a daikon radish and apply the gratings directly to the bruised area. Keep in place for twenty to thirty minutes with a clean dressing. Continue this once or twice a day as needed. Radish juice can also be used for this complaint

Fighting body odour

Body odour is caused when bacteria feed on sweat and in the process of breaking sweat down and digesting it cause chemicals to be released. It's these chemicals that are responsible for the unpleasant and all too familiar odour.

Radishes can help to fight body odour when used as a juice. After bathing or showering pat the armpits and feet dry, and then apply a handful of radish juice under each armpit, or onto the feet and in between the toes as necessary. Repeat this daily until the body odour no longer occurs.

Conclusion

I am rather fond of this vegetable, despite the fact that my introduction to it as a child caused me some distress. I wasn't prepared for the peppery flavour when I first bit into it, and certainly wasn't prepared for the telling off I received when I got caught using radishes from the allotment as playthings. Still, all is forgiven and the radish and I are best of friends.

To this effect radishes really are more than just a good salad ingredient. As you've seen they are useful for relieving common minor ailments, and with regards cleansing the palate before a glass of wine, well, I'm off now to give that a try – Santé.

ROLLING PIN

Picture the scene. An angry wife chasing her husband with a rolling pin, or a cook chasing food predators from her kitchen furiously waving the rolling pin in the air. It's very familiar isn't it? We've all laughed at this comedy creation and no doubt all used a rolling pin for its true function, to flatten dough. But how many have used it to sort out minor health complaints? Well, it's helpful for treating some of those too.

About rolling pins

Rolling pins come in many different shapes and sizes but there are two basic types. The more common roller is perhaps the type that most people are familiar with having a thick cylindrical centre with handles at each end to hold when using. It is made from a variety of materials, notably wood, but can also be from plastic and ceramic. The cylinder is usually 7–10cm in diameter and the handles are grasped to roll across the dough. Increasingly rolling pins are available in designs to accommodate the requirements of the most discernable cook or kitchen stylist. For example, the metropolitan stainless steel kitchen may have a stainless steel rolling pin, a brightly coloured kitchen a fluorescent coloured cylinder rolling pin, whilst the country kitchen might have a simple wooden rolling pin.

The other type of rolling pin is the rod or 'French' rolling pin. It differs from the roller in that it's a thin tapered baton, usually made of wood and used by placing the palm on the pin and rolling the rod across the dough. These usually have a diameter of 2–3cm, and fans of this type say that it allows the user to work the dough more easily.

Although rolling pins are mostly used to shape and flatten dough for biscuits, pie crusts, and pastries they can also be used for other culinary purposes. Nuts or biscuits placed in a sealed bag can be safely crushed with a rolling pin, and pieces of meat can be tenderised with one. If you are brave you can even crack eggs with a rolling pin.

Did you know?
In October 1920 *The American Woman Magazine* reported a way to use a rolling pin to improve the appearance of the neck. It suggested holding the rolling pin in both hands, and whilst holding it horizontal pushing it gently up against the chin.

Rolling pin history

Preparing and inventing dishes was popular with the Etruscans who lived in Ancient Italy and Corsica, around the Ninth Century BC. To assist them with their passion they developed tools, one of which was the rolling pin. This technology was passed on to the Romans, Greeks, and on into Europe where the rolling pin is an essential part of any kitchen.

It was only in the Nineteenth Century that rolling pins began to be factory produced. Up until that time rolling pins were made with whatever materials, and craft skills, were available. Smoothed tree branches and baked clay were early types. As time moved on glass bottles, ceramics, marble, and more recently stainless steel would be used.

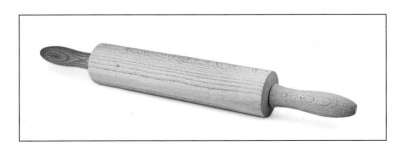

"Great for rolling out health problems too"

Many kitchen tools hold a personal value to an individual. This might be because despite its age the rolling pin always feels comfortable and makes achieving the desired outcome an effortless process, or because it's been handed down from one generation to the next and so holds sentimental value. In fact, rolling pins would often be personalised with individual designs that were created and commissioned and which included shapes and emblems carved into the wooden handles. Pottery rolling pins often had decorated cylinders with Delft-type windmills being popular designs. Glass rolling pins were often embossed with nautical emblems, presumed to have been created by sailors. Glass factory workers are said to have used left-over glass to make rolling pins that they then offered as gifts to loved ones, or someone they wished to court. Those glass rolling pins may have had a cap at one end to allow it to have a second role as a storage container. Edward Turleig described these, 'As love-tokens to be hung in the kitchen while Jack was at sea; as clandestine containers for rum or tea smuggled to avoid duty; as convenient containers for sugar.'

Marble rolling pins may be cooled in the refrigerator, and hollow rolling pins may be filled with water and would often be used to store essential cooking ingredients such as baking powder or vinegar. When emptied, filling the hollow cavity of the rolling pin with ice or cold water allowed the dough to be kept cool and at a better working temperature.

Rolling pin remedies

- **Aching feet** – The gentle action of massage can soothe aching feet and with a rolling pin is a simple way to achieve this. First soak feet in warm water for ten to fifteen minutes. Dry thoroughly. Whilst sitting place each foot in turn on the rolling pin, or together if the pin is long enough, and roll the pin forwards and backwards using your feet
- **Mastitis** – A painful condition that particularly occurs in breast-feeding women. The rolling pin can be used to bruise the veins of cabbage leaves before applying these, warmed, to the sore breast
- **Snoring** – Although the temptation may be to poke or hit the snoring person with the rolling pin there is a more appropriate, and kinder, use for it. Snoring is worse when lying on the back so placing the rolling pin next to the person whilst they are sleeping on their side, means if they try to roll onto their back they are discouraged from doing so because the presence of the rolling pin makes this uncomfortable. If the rolling pin should move then putting it inside the pyjama top, loose or sewn in, will overcome this
- **Cellulite** – Some report that massaging cellulite with a rolling pin lessens its appearance
- **Stress** – Making sure that there is nobody and nothing breakable or of value around, beat a pillow with the rolling pin. This is a way of relieving stress without causing further stress or harm

---

Fighting back pain

Back pain is a very common problem and is mostly caused by muscular injury. A rolling pin is a simple and effective tool to perform gentle back massage with. Ideally ask someone else to massage your back with the rolling pin but if this is not convenient it should be possible to do it yourself. Whilst standing with legs slightly apart, hold the rolling pin handles and roll it up and down the sore area to bring relief.

Conclusion

The first thing that comes to mind if you're a cook when thinking about a rolling pin is flattening dough and flour dust. If not, then it's a furious person, usually a woman, with her apron flapping, as she chases someone from her kitchen, usually bringing a smile to our face.

As you've seen it's not only through comedy that the rolling pin can bring smiles. It can bring these when it helps to relieve minor ailments too. There's bound to be at least one in your kitchen, usually within arm's reach. And remember, when using the rolling pin for its true purpose, the activity of rolling out the dough counts towards the day's activity quota, so make sure you put in some effort!

SALT

It's all around us and essential for everyday human life. Not only do our bodies depend on salt, but salt also plays an important part in food preservation and preparation too. Salt's benefits don't end there though as salt can be a useful thing to have around when minor ailments appear. We may add a pinch here, and a pinch there whilst cooking, but a pinch of salt may take us that little bit further on our road to recovery from troublesome health complaints.

About salt

Here's the science. The two major components of salt are sodium and chloride, in a ratio of forty per cent sodium to sixty per cent chloride. The body needs sodium to help regulate and maintain correct fluid balance, or water content, within it. It draws water in like a chemical sponge therefore stopping tissues in the body from becoming too dry. Sodium is also necessary for nerve impulse transmission and muscle contraction. The downside of sodium is that it contributes to high blood pressure, which is why in recent years campaigns have tried to raise awareness of this, and the fact that the average adult consumes far more, an estimated fifty per cent or more, each day than is needed. Around eighty per cent of the salt we consume is in food, which is why it's important to be aware of the fact that often it is sodium content that's listed on food packaging, and that to get the actual salt content you need to multiply the sodium value by 2.5.

The table salt that we are most familiar with is ninety-nine per cent sodium chloride, the remaining one per cent being made up of substances that prevent the grains of salt from sticking together allowing free flow of salt – you've seen damp salt in a salt cellar no doubt. In my experience salt cellars don't appear to be so common on tables these days? Perhaps that's because people are becoming more health conscious or because my family and friends know I'm coming and hide the salt cellar away! But the truth is a pinch of salt does add flavouring to food when cooking, and even I find it hard not to have salt on my bag of chips. When being asked to cut down on salt people are often worried about how food will taste, that it will taste, well, tasteless. It's true that initially food may not taste the same because taste buds get used to the flavour of salt but after around three weeks they will adapt to the new flavours, the true flavours of the food you eat. If you're still concerned black pepper, chilli, garlic, and herbs make good alternative seasonings.

Did you know?

People have 'taken the water' for years, and still do so. In France it is still a very popular therapy and those with the skin condition psoriasis often report improvements in their skin when it has been bathed in seawater. Some are fortunate to be able to travel to the Dead Sea where the high mineral and salt content of the sea water – the salt content is thirty-three per cent, compared with the ocean salt content of three per cent – is thought to contribute to the therapeutic effects. Salt water is very soothing for prickly heat too.

Salt history

Thousands of years ago salt was used as a preservative of foods, after all, the modern appliances we take for granted these days were not around – the first known artificial refrigeration was demonstrated in 1748 by William Cullen at the University of Glasgow.

Salt was traditionally also a sign of wealth and hospitality. It was offered as payment for goods or services, or given as a gift. The Roman Army troops were paid in salt and this gave rise to the word we are so familiar with today, salary.

The word salad originated from the process of salting leaf vegetables and actually means 'salted'. In the past having salt available to a guest indicated that the guest was valued and welcome to the household. Of course in modern times the presence of the salt cellar on a table is there for a person to add additional flavouring to a meal. In the past adding salt to the served food was a gracious acknowledgement of the host's generosity. Nowadays, the same behaviour may result in causing offence to the cook.

A trip to the seaside makes us feel good for a number of reasons – the fresh, often bracing

"A generous healer"

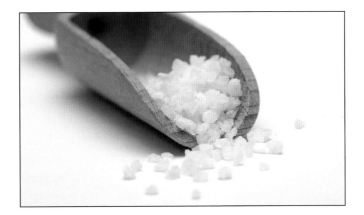

sea air, the open spaces, the familiar sounds of gulls and waves, and of course, a bag of chips covered in salt. With regards health for many years people have gone to the sea to gain the benefits of seawater cures. Not only does a dose of sea air clear the nasal passages but the many trace elements in seawater are felt to be beneficial to health. For example, manganese, copper and magnesium are thought to be able to relieve, and indeed prevent, nasal symptoms such as congestion, running, and swelling as they are believed to have anti-allergy and anti-inflammatory actions.

Salt remedies

- **Sore throat** – One of the most well-known home remedies making use of salt is to relieve a sore throat. Mix a third of a level teaspoon of salt into a cup of warm water. Gargle this half a dozen times, three or four times day. Do not swallow mixture
- **Genital infections** – Cystitis and genital infections such as herpes can be very painful making passing urine, and even just sitting down, very uncomfortable indeed. Bathing in salt water brings great relief. Add a tablespoon of salt to a bath of warm water, climb in and relax. For those having difficulty passing urine because of the pain, sitting in a salt water bath to pass urine makes this easier
- **Nasal congestion** – Make a mixture of two cups of warm water and half a teaspoon of salt. Apply this to the nasal passages on a cotton bud soaked in the mixture, or by using a dropper to squirt mixture into the nose. Another way to administer this remedy is to sniff the solution from a small glass into the nostril whilst closing the other nostril with your thumb
- **Mouth ulcers** – Placing salt directly against the ulcer helps relieve swelling and pain. Alternatively make a solution of a cup of warm water with a third of a level teaspoon of salt and rinse around the mouth, spitting it out afterwards
- **Pimples** – Salt can help to lessen swelling and redness. Mix one cup of warm water with one third teaspoon of salt. Soak a cotton bud or piece of tissue in the mixture and apply to the pimple. Vinegar can be added to this mixture if desired

- **Joint pains** – Heat salt in a pan and then make into a poultice. Place this against the sore joint
- **Chilblains** – Relieve inflammation of a chilblain by rubbing brandy and salt over the affected area. Alternatively, mix a few handfuls of salt in hot water. When at a comfortable temperature bath the feet or hands. Vinegar can be added to this if desired

Fighting ear problems

Blocked ears are commonly due to an accumulation of wax. Poking around with a cotton bud, or anything else for that matter should be avoided as doing this just makes it harder for the wax to come out, and may damage the ear canal. Softening the wax helps it come out naturally. Do this by adding salt to warm water and provided the water is not too hot gently irrigate the ear canal using a dropper or a teaspoon. For earache try making a poultice of warmed salt and placing this over the outside of the ear.

Conclusion

So a pinch of salt can make a great deal of difference to the food we eat and our health. Remember how consuming too much salt, as many people still do, can contribute to high blood pressure that in turn makes heart attacks and strokes more likely. However, clearly salt is beneficial when it comes to treating minor ailments, so whatever else you have in your kitchen, make sure there's a little salt, the only rock that we humans eat.

TEA BAGS

As I'm writing this the tea bag has just celebrated its one hundredth birthday, so in its honour I'm having a cup of tea, made with a tea bag of course. Not that I need an excuse because I've always enjoyed a nice cup of tea in the morning, and a nice cup of tea in the afternoon. In fact, thinking about it I enjoy it anytime. In the 1970s an advert proclaimed Martini as the drink for 'any time, any place, anywhere'. Well, for me they might have been describing a cup of tea as this provides a refreshing drink, a natural short break, and of course tea has protective health benefits too. Moreover, the tea bag can be put to very good use in treating common ailments.

About tea bags

For years there's been debate within my family, and I'm sure amongst other families too, about the cup of tea made with a tea bag not being as good as that made with loose tea leaves. I know when I was growing up to me it was a real palaver making a cup of tea as it needed loose leaves, a strainer, and goodness knows what else. On reflection however, this time taken making tea was therapeutic. You could argue that in our rushed lives perhaps we lose out a little because of the convenience of the tea bag as it can mean we don't get to spend so much time waiting for the tea to be ready and consequently miss out on a relaxing tea break. However, when you make a cup of tea with a tea bag you still have a chance for a break. In fact, a doctor I used to work with would often be heard, when giving a patient advice over the phone, to say, 'Now, I want you to make a cup of tea, and if you're not feeling better after drinking it, please call me again.'

The antioxidants in tea, called flavonoids, are thought to help keep the heart and circulation healthy and possibly to help reduce the risk of cancers. Certainly it contributes to our daily fluid intake requirement, and the caffeine can help boost our levels of alertness and concentration. A natural source of fluoride tea can help protect against gum disease and tooth decay. All in all, tea is felt by the majority of people to be good for us.

Nowadays tea bags come in many different shapes – circular, pyramids, and of course the traditional square bag that can usually be found in my briefcase. I try to make sure I always have a bag available, after all, you only need a cup or mug, some boiling water, and a dash of milk, and there you are.

Did you know?
In Britain it's estimated that 130 million cups of tea are consumed everyday, and that ninety-six per cent of these are made using tea bags.

Tea bag history

With its reputation as a nation of coffee drinkers you may be surprised to learn that tea bags originated in the United States, and like many great discoveries, by accident. A New York coffee merchant called Thomas Sullivan was struggling to reduce his business costs and decided to send samples of tea in small silk bags rather than loose. Those receiving the sachets didn't realise they were supposed to empty the contents into a pot and simply put the sachet in instead. All was fine, except that the silk mesh was too fine, so bags became made of gauze. Ten or more years later these first purpose-made tea bags became commercially produced, in two sizes, a larger bag for the pot and a smaller one for the teacup. A string and tag were added to make it easier to remove. Nowadays, modern tea bags are usually made from paper fibre.

We Brits were suspicious of this development, not enthusiastic about rumours that the bag should be dunked into a cup of lukewarm hot water. Let's be honest, only biscuits should be dunked! Although World War 2 held up the introduction of tea bags into the UK, Joseph Tetley drove their introduction in 1953, and was soon followed by other companies who recognised a growing acceptance and demand for modern convenience products. Now, of course, only the diehard tea drinkers refuse to entertain the tea bag. In fact, when recently

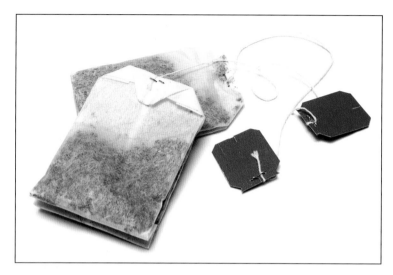

"You can't beat a nice cuppa"

visiting my aunt, I shudder to say this, but I noticed a container of tea bags on the shelf. Now that's something I never expected to see.

Tea bag remedies

- **Puffy eyes** – Using a tea bag can help to reduce puffiness. It's thought that the tannin in tea, a natural astringent, can help to reduce puffiness by pulling the skin taut. Add a tea bag to boiled water, leave for around five minutes and then remove the tea bag. Squeeze it out and allow it to cool to a tolerable temperature and then place over the puffy area and leave for ten to fifteen minutes. If you enjoy cold 'builder's tea', drink the tea afterwards

- **Foot odour** – Steep four tea bags in one or two pints of boiling water for twenty minutes. Transfer to a bowl large enough for your feet. Once cool enough to tolerate bathe both feet for thirty minutes. Repeat each night before retiring to bed

- **Stye** – Wet a tea bag and place over the stye and leave for a few minutes. The tannin in the tea is thought to help reduce the size of the stye

- **Sunburn** – Steep four tea bags in boiling water for ten minutes. Allow to cool, and then apply liquid to sunburned area using a cloth. Bites and stings can be eased with this remedy too

- **Chapped lips** – Soak a tea bag in warm water and press against lips for two to three minutes. Alternatively place a soaked tea bag in the refrigerator to cool and then apply to lips

- **Corns / calluses** – Moisten a tea bag and then tape against the corn or callus. Leave in place for thirty to sixty minutes. It may be more convenient to do this and leave it overnight. This remedy can be used to treat warts too

- **Minor bleeding** – Using a tea bag soaked in water apply this with light pressure to the bleeding area

- **Sore throat** – Add four to six tea bags to boiling water. Leave to steep for ten minutes, then allow to cool to a comfortable temperature to enable the liquid to be gargled but not swallowed

Fighting cold sores

Cold sores are uncomfortable and cause a great deal of misery. Tea bags have been used to treat them for many years and people report that they work. Soak a tea bag in hot water for about five minutes then remove it, squeeze it out, and allow it to cool so that it can be comfortably applied to the cold sore. Some people find that cooling the soaked tea bag in the refrigerator brings relief too. Repeat this as needed. This remedy can also be used to ease the pain of mouth ulcers. Earl Grey tea bags are also thought to work well because they contain bergamot oil, which may help healing.

Conclusion

There's so much goodness, and so many benefits to be had from this unassuming small and compact package. How lucky we are that the initial suspicions and resistance of our ancestors to the tea bag were overcome. Perhaps the tea bag was seen as a modern day Trojan horse? Well, if it was, it brought good as far as I'm concerned.

When someone asks me how I like my tea, I reply as it comes, because this is true and also if someone is kind enough to make me a cup, then I'm not going to be fussy. In fact, I've just been offered a cuppa, so I guess this is as good a time as any to sit back, feel the warmth in my hands, and do myself some good.

THYME

To smooth the passage of time, whether this is during illness or when on a journey of discovery, you may not need to look further than the well-known herb thyme. It's a herb that's associated with strength, courage and energy. For centuries it has been used for culinary purposes where it's still extensively used today. In days gone by before the advent of modern medicine it was widely used to treat many different common ailments, something it can still help do today.

About thyme

I'm sure you're very familiar with thyme and its association with cooking. For me it's a herb I mostly associate with adding flavour to lamb dishes. A component part of the 'bouquet garni' in French cuisine, alongside parsley and bay, it appears in dishes of many different cultures where in addition to being used to flavour meat dishes it also adds flavour to stews, soups, and stuffing.

Thyme is the herb of courage, its name being derived from the Greek word 'thumus', signifying courage. Traditionally, thyme was also seen as a herb bringing great advantage and approval. Despite how this comment might first have been interpreted, in Greek times being said 'to smell of thyme' was actually a compliment, being an expression offered to those whose style was thought to be graceful and elegant.

You may not be aware, however, that thyme has wide-ranging medicinal properties. It contains a substance called thymol that is a powerful antiseptic. Before the advent of antibiotics this was extensively used to treat infections of the skin, and was, and still is, added to dressings for this purpose. It can also help to treat fungal infections such as athlete's foot and is still added to a number of other medicinal products, for example mouth washes.

Did you know?

During the Middle Ages when a knight was setting off on a crusade his beloved would give him some thyme as a gift, which may have been sewn onto her scarf. The mere presence of thyme was believed to provide courage, but if eaten was said to offer even greater courage, and make the knight more daring – in battle presumably.

Thyme history

Thyme has always been held in high regard, arguably you could say it's a member of herb royalty. In Egyptian times it was used in embalming and not only did the Greeks use it to

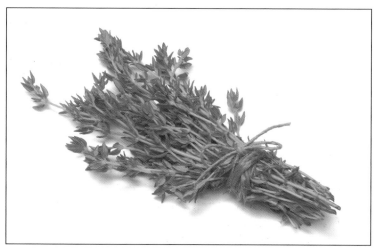

"Thyme is the healer"

compliment those they found stylish, but they also used it as incense in their temples because of their belief that thyme brought strength, courage, and protection.

The Romans made even more practical use of thyme, using it as incense to freshen up rooms. It was at this time that it's thought thyme began its role for culinary purposes, being used to add flavour to wines and cheese. Roman soldiers also made use of thyme being said to bathe in thyme water in order to become re-energised.

In essence thyme was regarded as making life easier, and the passage through life, and indeed death, a smoother one. It was put into coffins to gain passage to the next life, and was placed under pillows to aid sleep, prevent nightmares, and ward off evil beings. On a lighter note it was worn during the Middle Ages by the rich to ward off bad smells and germs from the poor.

Thyme remedies

- **Mouthwash** – Thyme can help to relieve toothache and sore gums, and can freshen breath. In fact it is included in some commercial mouthwashes today. Make a cup of thyme tea by infusing a sprig of thyme in hot water, and once cool enough rinse around the mouth as needed. This can be refrigerated to gain additional soothing benefit
- **Spots / boils** – Thyme is a powerful antiseptic so can be used to treat minor skin ailments such as boils, minor burns, and other minor wounds. Apply cooled thyme tea directly to the affected area or by using a clean cloth soaked in the tea. Thyme tea can also be applied to a clean dressing, which is then applied to the affected area. Where possible the affected part can be bathed in thyme tea. A tincture may also be made and applied a few times a day
- **Athlete's foot** – Apply thyme tea tincture a few times a day. Alternatively make sufficient thyme tea to fill a bowl large enough to put both feet in, and rest the feet in the tea at as hot a temperature as can be tolerated
- **Fever** – Make a thyme tea compress and place against the forehead
- **Sore eyes** – Make a compress of thyme tea and place gently over closed sore eyes. Leave for five to ten minutes
- **Sore throat and colds** – Thyme tea makes a very effective gargle to relieve a sore throat and irritating cough. Allow tea to cool to a temperature that can be tolerated then gargle the liquid. Do this as often as needed

Aching joints and muscles
Dried thyme herb can be very soothing for aching and tired joints and muscles. Add a few handfuls to a bath of warm water and then soak and relax in this. Alternatively, when filling the bath wrap a handful of dried thyme in a muslin bag and tie beneath the tap allowing water to flow through it. This can also be used

when showering. If it's not convenient to bath or shower make thyme tea, allow to cool, soak a clean cloth in it, and apply to affected area for ten to fifteen minutes.

Conclusion

I find it absolutely fascinating how thyme's role as a giver of courage and provider of protection has continued through the ages. Throughout the centuries thyme has been regarded as a protector of all things important and as a defence against many things bad, and continues to do so since even today it is recognised by many as offering similar benefits. For instance, it's actually quite an effective insect repellent, and with regards treating infection, its antiseptic properties are still employed.

Moreover, it has been regarded as something good, something that is associated with being pleasing on the eye, and indeed on the nostrils. In modern medicine I've often had to tell a patient that where no specific treatment is available for their condition, time is the healer. In future, perhaps I'll have to be more specific.

TOMATO

Is it a fruit, is it a vegetable, no it's super-tomato. Whatever the academics may argue one thing is for sure, tomatoes are good for us in so many ways. Bright red and cheerful, delicious to eat, tomatoes also promote self-confidence in the vegetable patch. At least, for me they do because they are one of the foods I've always succeeded in growing. Not only that, they are good for your health.

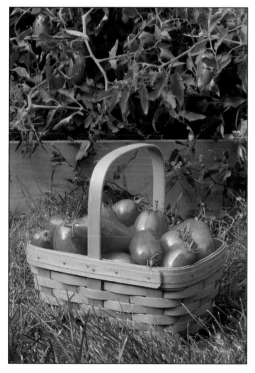

About Tomatoes

It's not easy to list all the many different ways tomatoes contribute to the foods we enjoy. Quickly, off the top of my head, and whilst having a look around my kitchen I've come up with the following – sauces, puree, paste, ketchup, casseroles, salad, chutney, relish, salsa, and what my daughter is making at this precise moment – pizza! Later on I may have a glass of tomato juice with Worcester sauce

"Throw these at minor ailments to get results"

to celebrate completing this chapter but in the meantime it's a delicious tomato sandwich that I'm going to enjoy.

Tomatoes vary in size and colour. If size matters to you then at one end of the scale we have the cherry tomato, at the other the beefsteak tomato that can be over ten centimetres in diameter. Most tomatoes though are somewhere in between. Although mainly red in colour this doesn't apply to all. Green, purple, orange and pink tomatoes are available, even multi-coloured and striped tomatoes exist. So there's something for everyone.

As for our internal health tomatoes often appear in lists of 'super foods' because they are rich in vitamins A and C, flavonoids and in carotenoids (which give them the bright red colour) and that are powerful antioxidants – substances that neutralise free radicals produced in the body as a normal part of metabolism but if left unchecked contribute to diseases such as heart disease, arthritis, and cancers. Something particularly special in tomatoes is lycopene, a carotenoid that is said to be one of the most powerful antioxidants. And of course, tomatoes provide us with dietary fibre too.

Did you know?

The carotenoid lycopene in tomato is thought to be protective against prostate cancer. Of note, however, is that cooking tomatoes actually increases the absorption of lycopene into the body, which is interesting as often it's the case that cooking vegetables decreases their nutritional value. Processed tomato products also contain higher concentrations of lycopene so another reason to not feel guilty about consuming tomato ketchup and baked beans, and for me in a moment, pizza!

Tomato history

The history of this wonderful vegetable has been full of misunderstanding and debate. Many say it originated in South America, in the Andes, and is believed to have first been cultivated by the Incas and the Aztecs as long ago as 700AD. Others argue it originated in Mexico. The Aztecs described the tomato well, giving it the name 'xitomatl', which means plump thing with a navel, a rather good description I think you'll agree, particularly as it was yellow in colour.

How it got to Europe is also unclear. Some believe Spanish conquistadors introduced it, as they did other foods from South America. Others believe the legend of two Jesuit priests bringing tomatoes from Mexico to Italy. Then there's the debate about whether the tomato is a fruit or a vegetable? In botanical terms it is actually a berry, making it a fruit, however, in culinary and nutrition terms it is thought of as a vegetable.

In France the idea that tomatoes may have aphrodisiac benefits is said to have arisen when a Frenchman misunderstood an Italian chef's description of the new ingredient in a meal the Frenchman had enjoyed. Described as 'Pomme de Maure' (Apple of the Moors) the Frenchman heard this as 'Pomme d'amour' (Apple of love) or love apple, which neatly takes us back to the plump thing with a navel!

For a long time tomatoes were thought of as being poisonous, partly because of their red colour being considered a danger, and partly because they belong to the deadly nightshade family. Of course, at least we're clear now that tomatoes are good and something to have around.

Tomato remedies

- **Skin** – The pulp of a tomato may help to tone and refresh the skin of the face. It can be made into a face pack by mixing tomato pulp with yogurt and applying to the face. Leave for around fifteen minutes then wash off. Rubbing the skin with fresh tomato a couple of times a day can lighten the skin if desired
- **Hangover** – A glass of tomato juice can help overcome a hangover, in fact taken before going to bed it may help prevent a hangover. It does this because vitamin C helps the liver process alcohol, the antioxidants help mop up free radicals, and liquid helps overcome dehydration that is responsible for the sandpaper mouth and woozy feelings
- **Sunburn** – Puree peeled tomatoes and add to a spoonful of yogurt or a spoonful of buttermilk and then apply to sunburn. Alternatively slice the tomatoes, dip in yogurt or buttermilk and apply to sunburn
- **Tired feet** – Ease the aching of tired feet by wrapping slices of tomatoes on the soles of the feet for twenty to thirty minutes. Alternatively place sliced tomatoes in an oval baking dish long enough to place feet in. Sit with feet resting on tomato slices for twenty to thirty minutes. If necessary you can use two dishes, one for each foot
- **Coughs and colds** – Tomato soup is something that I remember being given by my Mum when I was feeling poorly. It's the one thing I could eat. Since it has vitamin C, fluid to overcome dehydration, and is warming you can see how it might have helped. Anyway, it made me feel better, and that's half the battle

Fighting bad breath

For those who would like to be amorous, or simply don't want friends turning their nose at them, the tomato may help to overcome the problem of bad breath, medically called halitosis. This arises when in the process of feeding on food debris in the mouth bacteria release volatile sulphur compounds responsible for the odour of bad breath. Tomatoes are thought to contain compounds, for example, ionones that can convert these compounds into odourless ones.

Conclusion

It may be a vegetable that's often thrown when someone is unhappy but truly the tomato is a vegetable to be kept hold of, not discarded unceremoniously. A cheerfully coloured food, enjoyed in so many ways, for me it conjures up happy memories of relaxing summertime picnics in fields and by river banks. Moreover, knowing now about the health benefits means no one should feel guilty for enjoying processed tomato products.

If its colour doesn't make you smile, knowing it as your little plump thing with a navel will. Just be sure that if you call it that in public, you make it clear to those around you what you're talking about if you don't want to be on the receiving end of one!

TONIC WATER

Make mine a gin and tonic please. If I were to ask you to tell me a phrase that includes the word 'tonic' this one would probably come out top of the list, or at least, in a medal-winning position. Tonic water is one of those under-rated drinks in my opinion because we so often take it for granted, seeing it as perhaps the understudy to something else. It deserves a lime-light of its own though, so let's put it under the spotlight.

About tonic water

Everyone is familiar with tonic water. Well, most of us are. A wonderful refreshing drink that is comfortable with an accompanying partner, but also confident to stand alone. I remember a friend of mine relaxing back in a garden chair on a warm summer's evening and hearing him proclaim, 'Ah. A marriage made in heaven.' How lovely I thought to hear him say that about his relationship with his wife. It really summed up the evening we were having. Until I turned round from the barbecue I was supervising to find him romantically holding and gazing at a glass of gin and tonic.

Growing up I guess my impression, when I think back, of tonic water was as posh lemonade, or lemonade for grown-ups. After all, it's just carbonated water, flavoured with quinine, which is what gives

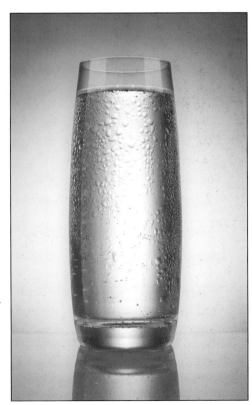

"One half of a perfect partnership"

it its bitter taste. As children we'd be offered lemonade, the adults would have tonic water, the ladies having slimline to try and keep the pounds off. I remember mum and dad making it themselves with a household tabletop gadget that pumped carbon dioxide into water – the 'Soda Stream' it was called. Perhaps it was the fun of pulling down the lever to introduce the gas, perhaps it was me wanting to be 'grown-up', or perhaps it was the taste, but I've always enjoyed the biting bitterness of tonic water. In fact, come to think of it I've always enjoyed bitter lemon too. I find these drinks refreshing, and a bit of a wake-up call.

Mention tonic water and some people will smile in recognition, not because of the association with alcohol, but because of using it to avoid night-time leg cramps. My grandmother swore by this, taking half a glass of tonic water – alone I should add – before bedtime to prevent being woken in the night with uncomfortable leg cramps. Tonic water, and specifically the quinine, has other benefits with regards treating health complaints, as we'll see.

Did you know?
Tonic water will fluoresce a blue colour under UV light. This is down to the quinine being sensitive to and excited by UV light. A good place to find this out is in a nightclub, now there's an excuse for you to go and party.

Tonic water history

Quinine is a useful muscle relaxant, and used for many years by the Quechua Indians of Peru to ease the muscle spasms that come with fever and infection. Quinine comes from the bark of the cinchona tree and this would be ground to a fine powder and added to liquid. Brother Agostino Salumbrino, a young apothecarist, observed them using quinine and sent a sample to Rome where malaria was prevalent in the swamps and marshes surrounding the city to test whether it could work to treat malaria.

A number of years later quinine was extracted from the South American cinchona tree bark and got its name from the Inca (Quechua) word for this tree bark 'Quina' meaning 'holy bark'.

It's said that tonic water actually began life as quinine water in the British colonies of India, in the seventeenth century. The medicinal quinine tonic was used to protect against malaria, endemic in those parts, and to treat fevers when these occurred. But its bitter taste was a problem. To overcome this hurdle gin and lemon juice was added to make it more palatable, easier to swallow you could say. A fondness for this drink developed and whether someone had a fever or not it was consumed and enjoyed, and the rest, as we say, is history.

As a note, although quinine is sometimes used to treat malaria drinking modern day tonic water is not recommended to prevent malaria as there simply isn't enough quinine in it, you'd have to drink loads of it. Moreover, nowadays there are modern anti-malarial treatments that are appropriate for different parts of the world.

Tonic water remedies

- **Pick-me-up** – This is one of my personal favourite uses for tonic water as it's a reviving drink and its bitter taste wakes me up and launches me into action
- **Arthritis** – Some people report a reduction in their symptoms of arthritis when drinking tonic water during flare-ups, and find that daily consumption helps keep symptoms at bay. It is thought that quinine may have some anti-inflammatory and painkilling effects. Up to a glass a day is unlikely to cause any harm
- **Coughs and colds** – A helpful drink to gain the possible anti-inflammatory, painkilling, and fever-reducing effects of quinine, plus its ability to relieve and prevent muscle spasms. Add some lemon if desired
- **Fever** – Quinine has a long history of being used to treat fever associated with infections. Drinking a glass of tonic water may help to lower high temperatures, and to help replace liquid that is lost from the body when it is fighting infection

Fighting night cramps

Probably the most recognised medicinal use for quinine nowadays, to relieve nocturnal leg cramps that are not just uncomfortable, and sometimes very painful, but also disturb sleep leaving a person tired the next day. Drinking up to a glass of tonic water before bedtime is a very effective remedy for preventing these cramps. Adding lemon helps to take the edge of the tonic water if its flavour is too bitter for the palate.

Conclusion

I don't know about you but all this talk of tonic water and its many interesting and beneficial uses has left me feeling a little dry in the mouth. I'm pretty sure I'm not going down with anything unpleasant so it must mean my body is telling me I need a little something to wet my whistle, as my Dad used to say. Which reminds me, I must ask him whether the Soda Stream is still in our family?

In the meantime, it's a little early for a gin and tonic, but a long glass of tonic water sounds very appealing at the moment. So, cheers.

TURMERIC

There are many foods and herbs that are said to have health benefits and have been used for centuries by people to treat a wide variety of ailments. Very few, however, make it into Western medicine and get taken seriously. One that has grabbed the attention and made people stop and think is turmeric, a herb that has made a successful transition from alternative to conventional medicine. Don't worry if you struggle to pronounce its name correctly,

I know I do. But if your kitchen doesn't have it you should think seriously about remedying this situation.

About Turmeric

You're bound to be familiar with turmeric in cooking, where it's notably used as a herb in curries providing a bitter and peppery flavour. You may even know that its yellow colour is used to provide colouring in other foods and dishes, for example, yellow cake and ice cream. But like me you may not have been aware that turmeric is sometimes used as a food additive to protect foods from sunlight. This last role is interesting because within the body turmeric is felt to have a protective role too, something that of late studies of the potential health benefits of turmeric have highlighted.

This herb that belongs to the ginger family, and is native to South Asia, has been creating quite a stir in Western medicine as it seems it can help no end of health complaints. Used for centuries in Ayurvedic medicine to treat minor injuries of the skin of one form or another its benefits have been confirmed in some scientific research. For instance, it has anti-inflammatory effects believed to be because it acts in a similar way to modern-day anti-inflammatory drugs offering good explanation as to why it can relieve the joint pain and inflammation associated with arthritis.

The yellow colour of turmeric is down to polyphenols, chemicals found in plants that are believed to have antioxidant benefits in neutralising the free radicals that are produced in the body in response to normal metabolism, smoking, and UV radiation. If not dealt with free radicals, as their name implies, can cause havoc health-wise. The health benefits of turmeric are thought to be because of one such type of polyphenol, a curcuminoid called, yes, you've guessed it, curcumin, another word I struggle to pronounce correctly. This is said to have anti-inflammatory effects and anti-cancer properties where it is believed to induce the death of cancer cells. This is in addition to its antioxidant benefits. And that's not all. It may be able to aid in the fight against Alzheimer's disease by preventing the plaque

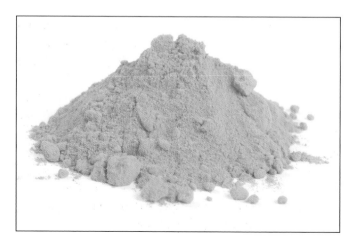

"A herb that's been making itself known"

formation responsible for this disease in the brain, and may be able to break up existing plaques.

So, it's an exciting time for this humble herb.

Did you know?

Turmeric may also help to deter ants. It's not known exactly how but anecdotally sprinkling a line of turmeric around the area prevents the ants from entering. It's that protective role again.

Turmeric history

Turmeric is believed to have most probably originated from Western India, where it has been used for 2,500 years or more. Its journey took it to China, across East to West Africa, and by the Eighteenth Century to the Caribbean.

Initially it is thought to have been used as a dye before it found its way into foods. Widely used as an inexpensive alternative to the more expensive saffron, in medieval Europe it became known as Indian Saffron.

In India turmeric, commonly known as Haldi in the Hindi language, is highly respected. It plays an important part in Hindu marriages where it's made into a paste with honey and almond oil and applied to the skin to nourish and purify it.

Now of course the whole world has heard of turmeric, and its potential health benefits are the focus of large amounts of research.

Turmeric remedies

- **Ringworm** – Make a paste by mixing two tablespoons of turmeric into boiling water. Add one tablespoon of lemon or lime juice if desired. Apply paste to the affected areas with a clean cloth and leave for twenty to thirty minutes. Hold in place by taping the cloth or by using cling film if possible. Do this twice a day
- **Joint pains** – Turmeric is probably best known for its anti-inflammatory effects and can be put to good use to relieve painful joints and muscles. Make a paste as above and apply to the affected area, fixing in place with cling film, or a dressing. This can also be used to treat muscle strains
- **Earache** – Mix a pinch of turmeric powder with a pinch of baking soda and carefully place in the outer part of the ear canal. This helps to dry up any discharge and calm down any inflammation. Do not push into the ear
- **Sore itchy skin** – Mix together coconut oil with turmeric powder and gently apply to the affected area. This can help to treat eczema, psoriasis, and bites and stings
- **Pimples and sores** – The discomfort and itch of sores caused by genital herpes and chickenpox can be eased by mixing turmeric powder with coconut oil, or by mixing turmeric powder with lime juice and water, and applying to the sores

- **Sore throat** – Into a cup of boiling water mix half or one teaspoon of turmeric powder and then gargle the mixture. Do this as needed

Fighting haemorrhoids

Haemorrhoids are usually the result of straining on the toilet and can be painful and itchy. The anti-inflammatory effects of turmeric can be put to good use to ease the discomfort. Make a paste by mixing two tablespoons of turmeric into boiling water. Add one tablespoon of lemon or lime juice if desired. Apply paste to haemorrhoids and hold in place for twenty to thirty minutes with a clean cloth by taping if possible. If not, sit on it. Do this twice a day. Turmeric can also be used to stop bleeding, something that can occur with haemorrhoids.

Conclusion

Talk about into the limelight, that's where turmeric now is. Of course, in some parts of the world it's always been regarded as one of the best, if not the best, herbs to have around for what it adds to cooking and healing.

Turmeric exemplifies how effectively foods can be used to help treat minor ailments, and how foods can help to keep us healthy, as modern science is proving. Yellow is a cheerful colour, it makes us feel good, so yet another benefit of this simple spice.

So, if you'll forgive the misuse of the words of the Bard, 'Turmeric or not turmeric, in your kitchen, that is the question.' The answer? Well, there is only one answer in my mind.

VINEGAR

Would you like salt and vinegar with that? Depending upon how virtuous I'm feeling at the time, or how guilty I'm feeling for that matter, the answer may be yes, or no, to this well-known chip shop enquiry. When it comes to having vinegar available at home the answer is always a resounding yes. After all, there are lots of uses for vinegar, treating minor ailments effectively being one of these.

About vinegar

Off the top of my head I can count dozens of uses for vinegar and I'm sure you can too. To keep things simple though the categories of cooking, cleaning, and cures, are what immediately spring to mind.

Yes, of course vinegar is used in food preparation, commonly in the process of pickling, and also in making salad dressings such as vinaigrettes. It's also added as a condiment to food such as the British favourite fish and chips, and used as an ingredient in ketchup – also added to fish and chips in my house – mayonnaise, and mustard. Let's not forget what is often a child's first, and often surprising, introduction to vinegar, and I think may actually have been mine, salt and vinegar crisps where vinegar is used as a flavouring.

Vinegar gained its name from the French 'vin aigre', meaning sour wine, and can be made by oxidation of practically any liquid that contains alcohol. There are many different varieties with white, malt, and apple cider being common ones.

Vinegar is a popular cleaner too traditionally being put onto newspaper and used to clean glass surfaces such as mirrors. Mixed with table salt vinegar can return stained cookware to its previously stainless appearance. Pouring baking soda down a drain, followed by a vinegar chaser, leaving this to work for five to ten minutes then finishing off the job with hot water helps prevent build-

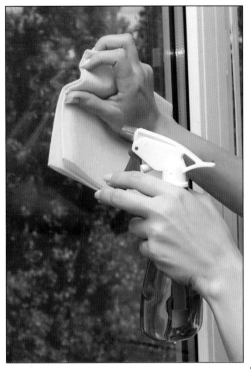

"When I'm cleaning windows"

up. Cover the drain whilst the baking soda and vinegar are getting acquainted because remember chemistry classes and how these two form a somewhat eruptive relationship.

Did you know?
You can stop a cat from scratching furniture by spraying white distilled vinegar onto the furniture. Also vinegar is very helpful for removing chewing gum from clothes if it's rubbed onto the gum before washing. A bowl of vinegar also helps remove fresh paint smells from a room.

Vinegar history

Vinegar has been utilised throughout history with traces having been found in Egyptian urns dating as far back as 3000BC. How it was discovered isn't precisely known. Some say it was probably by accident more than 10,000 years ago when the passage of time saw untouched wine turn sour. Then hey presto, vinegar was created.

With the passage of time vinegar has also found favour with many historical figures. Helen of Troy bathed in vinegar to relax, Caesar's armies drank vinegar, and Hannibal drenched heated boulders in vinegar cracking these into smaller rocks, enabling his army to cross the

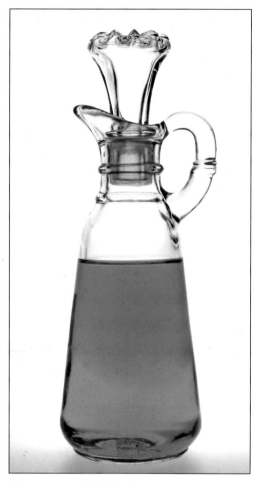

"So many uses, so little time"

Alps. In fact Cleopatra also demonstrated the solvent power of vinegar by dissolving precious pearls in it to win a bet that she could consume a fortune in a single meal.

Vinegar also has a long history of use in medicine. Hippocrates prescribed vinegar to treat many ailments, and to protect themselves from infection during the Bubonic Plague people covered their skin with vinegar. During World War 1 it was used to treat soldiers' wounds making use of its antiseptic and antibacterial properties, and now in modern times it is still used to treat sore throats, dandruff, and irritated skin.

Vinegar remedies

- **Irritated skin** – A mixture of two tablespoons of vinegar with a cup of water will ease the discomfort of itchy skin caused by stings or sunburn, for example, when applied to the affected area. This mixture of vinegar and water makes a useful alternative to soap when itchy skin anywhere around the body, for example the rectal area or feet, is a recurrent problem
- **Bruises** – Apply cooled vinegar to the bruised area with a compress for ten to twenty minutes. Repeat this a few times during the day
- **Body odour** – Mix equal parts of apple cider vinegar and water then apply to the armpits daily, or to other parts of the body that are causing problems
- **Sore throat** – Mix one tablespoon of vinegar in warm water and then gargle to ease a sore throat. Add honey and lemon to this if desired, and swallow the mixture after gargling first. Growing up this was known as 'Dad's daily dose', which he gave to me before bedtime during the hayfever season to prevent me suffering night-time symptoms
- **Fungal infection** – Vinegar has some degree of anti-fungal benefit so can be used to treat athlete's foot, for example, or used to treat dandruff – often caused by fungal infection – by soaking the scalp and hair with vinegar, leaving for an hour or so, and then rinsing

- **Corns and calluses** – These can be softened by soaking the feet in a foot bath of warm water and vinegar for twenty to thirty minutes
- **Itchy ears** – Mix a teaspoon of vinegar with half a cup of water and with the head tilted to one side use a medicine dropper to put a few drops into the ear

---

Fighting aching joints

Many people report getting relief from aching joints when using vinegar. Some benefit from rubbing warmed vinegar into the affected joint. Others report improvement from consuming vinegar, particularly apple cider vinegar, on a daily basis.

Conclusion

It may be a sour wine but vinegar sure does have many benefits to be utilised around the home. It can be put to work in food preparation, cleaning, laundry, and in the garden too, where it can kill weeds and stop ants from getting together.

Of course, vinegar helps to get rid of many minor ailments and although much of its use in healthcare is based on anecdote, so are many of the home remedies that have been used over the years. So think about pouring that bottle of vinegar a little bit further than a bag of chips.

WITCH HAZEL

Hubble, bubble, toil and trouble may be a familiar part of a witch's spell but it certainly isn't what you get with the super plant that is witch hazel. Unique amongst its peers in so many ways witch hazel is one of those remedies that can bring so much benefit when dealing with common minor ailments.

About Witch hazel

Witch hazel is a wonderful plant for many reasons. Not only is it rather nice to look at but it also has a rare quality amongst trees that its flowers, fruit and the following year's leaf buds all appear at the same time. In fact, even its horticultural name, *Hamamelis virginiana*, reminds us about healthy living as these are taken from the Greek words meaning 'together' and 'fruit', often combined as 'together with fruit', which of course is what we should all be doing with our daily diet.

For many years witch hazel has been used to treat all manner of minor ailments: notably haemorrhoids, varicose veins, and sore and itchy skin resulting from eczema and burns for instance. It's for treating bruises that I first came across it a number of years ago. I have to say that when the person started to reach into her bag, mentioning quite casually that I needed some witch hazel for the bruise that was sure to appear on my shin, I wasn't entirely confident and suspected some home-made potion to come out of her home-knit bag.

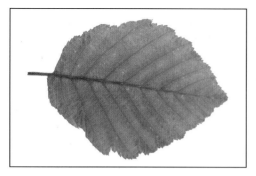

"All for one, and one for all"

However, time has moved on and witch hazel is now one of my firm favourites, confirming once again that you should never judge a book by its cover.

Witch hazel leaves contain substances called tannins and it's these that are thought to be responsible for its astringent property, and its ability to stop bleeding, in scientific terms called haemostasis. However, in the process of making witch hazel water or hamamelis water – most often found in commercial products, where to make this, recently cut twigs of the plant are soaked in warm water, steam distilled to release the essential oils, and alcohol added – tannins are lost, not appearing in the distillate which still has astringent properties. So clearly there are other chemicals present that contribute to these astringent effects. Buy hey, this is science and what I'm interested in is how it can help treat minor ailments.

Did you know?
In the past witch hazel was a favourite wood for dowsing, also known as water witching.

Witch hazel history

As with my first meeting with witch hazel you too could be forgiven for initially wanting to keep it at arms' length. After all, its name may conjure up an image of something to be wary of – most of us assume wickedness when we hear the word 'witch' don't we?

However, support it many people have done over the years. The American Indians certainly made good use of witch hazel in treating skin complaints, to soothe sore muscles, and as it is keenly used today, to treat cuts and bruises. Presumably it was witch hazel they reached for off screen after doing battle with cowboys in the legendary Western movies. John Wayne said, 'Get off your horse and drink your milk.' He wouldn't have been wrong to have said, 'Get off your horse and put some witch hazel on that.'

Early European settlers were introduced to the healing benefits of this medicinal plant by the aforementioned Native American Indians. Later in the Nineteenth Century herbalists introduced the preparation that commonly appears in commercial products, hamamelis water, made by distillation and the addition of alcohol.

Witch hazel remedies

- **Varicose veins** – The astringent tannins in witch hazel help to soothe varicose veins and temporarily tighten them, helping to relieve any discomfort and unpleasant appearance

- **Sore throat** – Witch hazel can help to soothe an irritating sore throat when used as a gargle. Using fresh witch hazel tea, made by boiling a handful of leaves for around five minutes and then straining, allow this to cool to a tolerable temperature and then gargle, spitting it out afterwards. This can also be used to treat sore and inflamed gums
- **Itchy skin** – A cotton wool ball or a clean cloth soaked in witch hazel tea and then applied to the affected area can soothe and reduce the inflammation of itchy and irritated skin
- **Bruises** – One of the most common uses for witch hazel is to apply witch hazel to the bruised part. This can be using tea, tincture, or a cream
- **Cold sores** – Daily application of witch hazel to the cold sore may help to speed up the recovery from these
- **Minor cuts** – The properties of witch hazel can help to stop bleeding from minor cuts. A few drops of a witch hazel tincture or decoction applied to the cut using a cotton bud is usually effective. This can be used to treat shaving nicks

Fighting haemorrhoids
Many commercially available products to treat haemorrhoids contain witch-hazel, making use of its anti-inflammatory and astringent properties. A simple way to use witch-hazel at home for this purpose is to soak a clean cloth in witch-hazel tea and apply this to the haemorrhoids two or three times a day for five to ten minutes. Witch-hazel tincture can be used as an alternative by applying a few drops of the tincture to the haemorrhoids using a cotton bud. This remedy can also be used daily to prevent haemorrhoids too.

Conclusion

Witch hazel branches are said to have helped people find their way to water in the past. Nowadays, the role of witch hazel has changed somewhat, but it's still a leading role it has to offer, and that is, leading us to soothing relief from the common ailments that come our way.

So, I hope you are ready to give witch hazel a chance to soothe and relieve the minor ailments that are likely to come your way at some time or another. Use it from scratch, have it ready prepared, or have a commercial product to hand. Which ever you choose, providing the Cub Scout's motto 'be prepared' is followed, problems should be nipped in the bud effectively.

YOGURT

I hope you enjoy yogurt as much as I do. It's played such an interesting part of my life for as long as I can remember, from helping me to get off to a good start at the beginning of the day, to seeing me comfortably through miles and miles of cycling in Europe. Of course, it's very popular in health circles for a number of reasons, which you're about to find out about.

About yogurt

This is one of my favourite foods. Forget the fact that it's now often considered a health food, I still regard it as a very enjoyable breakfast, snack, or dessert. I remember the days when only the 'Ski' yogurt pot with its distinctive shape appeared to be available but now of course there's an abundance of flavours and brands to choose from. Straightforward natural yogurt, fruit yogurt with pieces of fruit, or fruit blended in. This added, that added, something else added. Now there's frozen yogurt, and yogurt covered raisins and other dried fruits to enjoy too.

I believe there is truth in the healthy food claims. As a dairy product yogurt is an excellent source of calcium, vital for strong bones and teeth. It's also nutritionally rich in protein and some B vitamins. Nowadays it may also have probiotics added, the friendly bacteria our gut needs to function well.

Yogurt is produced by fermenting milk using harmless bacteria. During this fermentation process sugar produces lactic acid that in turn reacts with milk protein. The result is the characteristic creamy consistency of yogurt, and its tangy flavour. It's because of this sourness, that's often too much for some people, that fruit is added to sweeten it.

Thinking back, yogurt was one of the first natural remedies I was introduced to. One of my female patients wanted to share with me the wonderful way she had found to get rid of her thrush infection. Suffice to say, at the time I thought she was pulling my leg. Either that or she was, well how do I say, in need of some professional mental health intervention would be the medically accurate way of putting it. But, I was to learn that she had a point.

Did you know?

Many different countries have laid claim to the honour of inventing this popular food. However, it's said by some that yogurt originated in Turkey, when a pitcher of milk, belonging to a Turkish nomad, was contaminated with organisms that thrived in hot temperatures. This became known as 'yogurut', and subsequently many years later was called 'yoghurt', the name, and one of the spellings, we know it by today.

Yogurt history

It's thought to have originated in the Middle East, possibly as far back as 10,000BC where it's been a staple food for centuries. Clearly recognised for its health benefits for a long time – possibly since around 500BC – it was known as the 'Milk of eternal life'. In the latter half of the Twentieth Century yogurt was still being viewed by some as a fantastic health food. Its popularity in the United States took off further when it was heavily promoted as a health wonder food, helping people to look younger and live longer. Although no scientific evidence supports any anti-ageing claims it certainly is good for health helping maintain good bowel function and of course sufficient calcium in the body.

I will always have a fondness for yogurt. Not just because of its delicious flavour, wonderful refreshing texture, and nutritious value, of course. But because it saw me through some of my early travels in Europe, specifically, cycling around France in my gap year. Not having much money, or indeed much command of the French language, yogurt was one food that was readily and cheaply available. Moreover, it was available in family-sized pots, something I hadn't seen before – possibly because as a teenager visiting a supermarket wasn't high on my list of favoured activities. Anyway, I have happy memories of sitting on French kerbsides tucking into a family-sized strawberry yogurt pot, with the spoon of my Youth Hostel Association combination knife-fork-spoon set. Since I managed to travel around France, sleeping rough mostly, without suffering illness, I guess all those years ago without knowing it at the time I was introduced to the health benefits of yogurt.

Yogurt remedies

- **Bad breath** – Eating a daily portion of yogurt may help to eliminate and prevent bad breath. This is supported by some scientific research that suggests active bacteria in

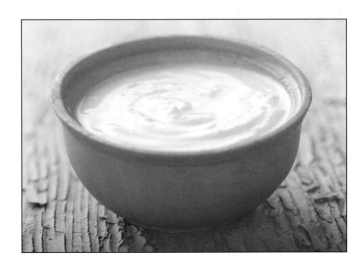

"This will see you through the good times, and the not so good times"

yogurt may inhibit the odour-causing bacteria in the mouth and so reduce levels of odorous hydrogen sulphide

- **Sunburn** – Yogurt is an effective way to relieve uncomfortable sunburn. It can be applied directly to the sunburnt skin or soaked in a cloth and dabbed onto the skin. Leave it to dry, and then rinse off with cool water
- **Razor burn** – Using plain yogurt gently apply to the sore area and leave to dry. Rinse off with cool water and then pat dry
- **Athlete's foot** – Yogurt is recognised as having anti-fungal benefits and so applying plain yogurt to the affected parts of the feet can help to treat athlete's foot. Alternatively, if you have enough plain yogurt, soak the feet in a bowlful
- **Dry skin** – Yogurt can be used to improve many different skin conditions including enlarged pores and dry skin. It can be applied directly to the skin, allowed to dry and left for ten to fifteen minutes, before being rinsed off with cool water. To moisturise the skin fresh cucumber can be pureed with plain yogurt and gently massaged into the skin, once again being left to dry and then rinsed off. Adding orange peel to plain yogurt, or oatmeal, makes it an ideal face scrub and skin exfoliator

Fighting thrush

Since I was introduced by one of my patients to the idea of using plain live yogurt to treat vaginal thrush, many more people have mentioned successfully treating their thrush with this therapy. In fact, even medical authorities no longer turn their nose up at the suggestion even though there's no conclusive scientific evidence to say it works. But how do you use it though? Well, some suggest consuming plain yogurt, but this is more likely to work in preventing recurrences. Putting plain live yogurt into the vagina is what most women do, using a tampon applicator to introduce the yogurt, which means more of the yogurt gets to where it needs to be, and of course, this way is less messy than other ideas I've heard about.

Conclusion

Yes, it's one of my favourite foods because it tastes so good, and by George it does me good. In fact, it helps both inside and out. It helps aid good digestion and gut function, and can be extensively used for skin ailments where it is useful not only as a moisturiser itself but also as a vehicle for other foods and substances when using these to treat skin conditions and improve the appearance of the skin. Yogurt comes in a convenient pot too, that afterwards can usually be recycled, or used for fun when making a whole host of children's toys.

So if you're not rushing out to make sure you've some yogurt in the fridge perhaps you should be? I suggest having two pots, one for eating, and one that's clearly labelled for health uses. Otherwise, what's likely to happen? Yes, you guessed it. When you need to reach for a handful of yogurt, there won't be any there, and that's not going to be helpful at all.

No longer used

Arsenic

The immediate reaction to the word arsenic is to conjure up an image of murder. After all, it's an effective killer of humans. For many years arsenic was the instrument of choice when wanting to be rid of someone because in large amounts it kills quickly, in smaller amounts it kills slowly causing, for instance headache, vomiting, abdominal pain, and liver and nervous system disorder. These non-specific symptoms meant the murderer could deflect any suspicion by suggesting these were due to a more likely, and less evil, explanation. Moreover, attending physicians would have drawn the same conclusion as until the time when a chemical test became available for arsenic it was impossible to conclusively prove that a person's demise had been at the hands of this poison.

In Victorian times women rubbed arsenic into their arms and face to improve their skin and complexion. It was also consumed, mixed with chalk and vinegar, by women to achieve paler facial skin and to create the perception of good breeding.

In the past arsenic compounds were used in medicines, for example to treat syphilis, but now is no longer used for this purpose and only used with great caution in the treatment of a type of leukaemia.

Mercury

It's gone out of fashion of late has mercury. This is primarily a consequence of the greater knowledge and understanding of its potential toxic effects. However, in the past it was extensively used in medicine.

In years gone by the Chinese believed that mercury healed fractures, maintained health and prolonged life. It's somewhat ironic that the First Emperor of China is said to have died as a result of trying to achieve eternal life by drinking a mixture of jade powder and mercury. The ancient Greeks made use of mercury in skin ointments, something also done by the ancient Egyptians and the Romans.

In medicine mercury was used as an internal cleanser making use of its laxative and diuretic effects. In fact in the Nineteenth Century mercury was the main ingredient in a treatment made in the United States called Blue mass, used to treat all manner of problems including constipation, toothache, depression, and the pain of childbirth. Mercury was extensively used as a disinfectant and to treat syphilis. In fact, as recently as the early part of the Twentieth Century mercury was being given to children in powdered form to treat teething pain, constipation, and worms.

Take a look around a doctor's consultation room and like in other medical establishments you'll find the traditional blood pressure measuring mercury sphygmomanometer and mercury thermometer have been superseded by electronic versions.

Formaldehyde

This is actually an effective disinfectant, and of course, a preservative, which is why formaldehyde-based products were used in embalming to temporarily fix and firm the tissue. In the past it was used extensively to kill bacteria but officially is no longer used for this purpose since modern equivalents have become available. It has been used over the years to treat warts where its effect is to dry the skin, and some would sniff it up the nostrils to treat a cold.

Exposure to formaldehyde can result in toxicity with symptoms of eye irritation, headache, throat discomfort that feels like burning, and the triggering of asthma and other allergic reactions. It also increases the risk of some cancers and for this reason in Europe its use has been banned.

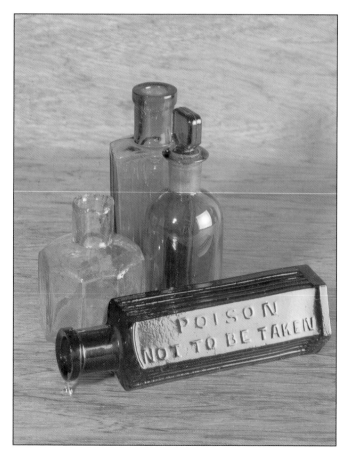

'Times have moved on'

Gin

It's a bit of a joke in my family, the use of alcohol to relieve, soothe, and calm down common ailments. I say joke, but what I mean is when I ask about remedies used when I was growing up, the question 'Was there ever any alcohol in that?' usually gets a smile and a reply along the lines of, 'Oh, I can't remember, it was a long time ago.'

Not so long ago, and probably still to this day although few people would admit to it nowadays, a small drop of alcohol was given to treat babies and children with colic and teething pain, for example. In fact, some commercial products for this purpose contained alcohol. Many people with arthritis still swear by eating gin-soaked raisins.

Alcohol is still one of the first remedies many people reach for when feeling stressed or a bit low, not that this is the best option because alcohol is a depressant and despite fooling someone in the short-term that things feel better, in the longer-term it makes matters worse.

Despite concern about alcohol consumption and the long-term harm it can have on the body, alcohol is still widely used externally as an antiseptic to clean wounds. Recently alcohol-based products have seen a resurgence in their popularity as they are increasingly used to help combat the spread of hospital-acquired infections such as MRSA.

Health Ailments

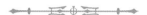

ACNE

This is a very common condition that usually starts in puberty. It's caused by sebaceous glands in the skin being oversensitive to testosterone and producing excess oily sebum. Stress makes it worse.

It is excess sebum and dead skin cells, not dirt, that block the hair follicles resulting in blackheads, which when inflamed become angry-looking red spots. Despite popular belief fatty foods do not cause acne.

Conventional treatment

Resist the temptation to pick the spots as doing this spreads inflammation and makes scarring more likely. Medicated lotions and face washes, creams and gels containing benzoyl peroxide, antibiotics and specific drugs for acne are used depending on how severe and widespread the acne is.

Old-fashioned remedies

- **Arnica** – Ready-made arnica cream can be applied to acne spots. Alternatively boil arnica flowers in water for five to ten minutes, strain the liquid and then apply to the acne spot using cotton wool once the liquid is at a temperature that the skin can tolerate
- **Bicarbonate of soda** – Apply a paste of bicarbonate of soda and water to the spots
- **Coconut oil** – Apply coconut oil to the affected area as required. Turmeric can be mixed with the coconut oil if desired
- **Cucumber** – Grate some cucumber and apply to the skin. Leave for about twenty minutes and then gently wash it off
- **Horseradish** – Add two tablespoons of grated horseradish to half a cup of honey and leave overnight. Apply the mixture three to four times a day with cotton wool to the affected skin until healed
- **Lemon juice** – Add one to two tablespoons of lemon juice to boiling water, allow to cool, then use the lemon and water mixture to cleanse the skin and spots

- **Onions** – Simmer one sliced onion with honey until soft. Make into a paste, allow to cool, then apply to the spot
- **Papaya** – Apply sliced, mashed, or as a juice by massaging into the skin and allowing to dry. Leave for five to ten minutes and then rinse off gently with cool or warm water
- **Salt** – Mix one cup of warm water with one third of a teaspoon of salt. Soak a cotton bud or piece of tissue in the mixture and apply to the spot. Vinegar can be added to this mixture if desired
- **Thyme** – Apply cooled thyme tea directly to the affected area or use a clean cloth soaked in the tea. A tincture may also be made and applied a few times a day
- **Turmeric** – Mix with coconut oil and apply to the spots

ALZHEIMER'S DISEASE

This is the most common form of dementia and is more likely as someone gets older.

It develops when deposits of protein kill brain cells disrupting the brain's normal function.

Over time a person loses their memory, gets confused, and may not recognise where they are or loved ones. Their personality may change and they may find it hard to communicate and do everyday things.

Conventional treatment

There's no cure but medication may help slow the deterioration. Memory therapy and other therapies such as occupational therapy often help, as does sticking to a routine. Gingko biloba may help maintain memory and prevent further deterioration.

Old-fashioned remedies

- **Lavender** – To help calm the mind and body add lavender essential oil to a pillow, pyjamas, or a handkerchief for daytime use. Inhaling the steam from a hot lavender infusion, drinking this, or adding lavender to a warm bath and soaking in this can help ease stress
- **Lemon balm** – Drinking warm lemon balm tea a couple of times a day can help lift someone out of depression

ANAL FISSURE

This is a tear in the skin just inside the back passage. Constipation and passing hard stools is a very common cause of an anal fissure, which bleeds and is very painful.

Conventional treatment

In a mater of weeks the anal fissure will heal of its own accord. Whilst this is happening painkillers and anaesthetic cream keeps things comfortable. Taking a stool softener, a gentle laxative, and eating more fibre makes passing stools easier and pain less likely. Eating plenty of fibre helps prevent it happening again.

Old-fashioned remedies

- **Calendula** – Apply as a cream or ointment or alternatively make an infusion of calendula leaves, soak a clean cloth in this, and apply to the affected area. It can be applied as a warm poultice too
- **Cloves** – Mix clove oil with yogurt and apply as a cream to the fissure
- **Honey** – After cleaning the area with water and patting it dry apply honey to a clean dressing and place the honey coated side of the dressing against the fissure
- **Lavender** – Make a lavender infusion using the flowers, strain and leave until the temperature is tolerable to the skin. Apply directly to the affected area or as a compress
- **Witch hazel** – Soak a clean cloth in witch hazel tea and apply this to the affected area two or three times a day for five to ten minutes. Alternatively apply witch hazel tincture using a cotton bud

ANXIETY

Feelings of anxiety can be normal, for example before a job interview or having to give a presentation. Anxiety becomes a problem when it is felt most of the time, and is severe enough to be affecting everyday life.

Anxiety can cause many symptoms including difficulty concentrating, feeling 'on edge',

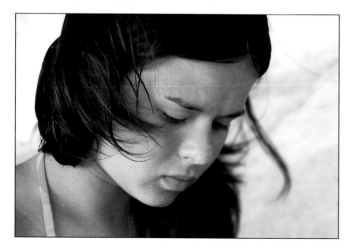

"Anxious times"

and a sense of dread. Physically it can cause a dry mouth, stomach 'butterflies, a need to go to the toilet often, palpitations, and problems sleeping.

Conventional treatment

Lifestyle measures such as regular exercise, reducing alcohol and caffeine consumption, not smoking all help as does practising relaxation techniques. Counselling and medication may be recommended.

Old-fashioned remedies

- **Camomile** – Drink a cup of camomile tea a few times a day to relieve stress and tension
- **Feverfew** – Drink a cup of weak feverfew tea or eat a few leaves in a sandwich
- **Lavender** – Add lavender essential oil to a pillow, clothing, or a handkerchief. Inhaling the steam from a hot lavender infusion, drinking this, or adding lavender to a warm bath and soaking in this can help ease stress
- **Lemon balm** – Drink a cup of warm lemon balm tea a couple of times a day

ARTHRITIS

There are many different types of arthritis with osteoarthritis being the commonest, caused by wear and tear of the joints. Other common types are rheumatoid arthritis and gout.

Arthritis causes joint inflammation, pain, swelling, and stiffness that can limit mobility. In turn this can make it hard for someone to maintain their independence.

Conventional treatment

This depends on the type of arthritis but will generally include painkillers and anti-inflammatory medication, exercise, physiotherapy, and sometimes surgery to replace a joint. For osteoarthritis glucosamine and chondroitin sulphate may be recommended.

Old-fashioned remedies

- **Arnica** – Apply a tincture of arnica to the affected joint or joints with a compress or poultice and fix to the joint with a bandage and leave for fifteen to twenty minutes
- **Basil** – Drink an infusion of basil twice a day
- **Bay leaf** – Tie leaves up in a small muslin cloth and soak in hot water, allow to cool, and then gently rub against the sore area. Alternatively, heat a handful of bay leaves in olive oil for fifteen to twenty minutes, allow to simmer for a further ten minutes, strain the oil, and rub against the affected area once cool enough to do so
- **Cabbage** – Place chilled cabbage leaves against the affected joint for a couple of hours.

Alternatively, warm up the leaves first by blanching in boiling water, running a hot iron over them, or putting them in a microwave

- **Feverfew** – Soak a clean cloth in a freshly brewed feverfew infusion and apply to the affected joint. If more than one joint is affected it may be simpler to consume a cup of weak feverfew tea
- **Figs** – Soak four figs in water and then mash these into a poultice. Apply directly to the affected area and keep in place with a clean cloth or dressing. Leave for thirty minutes to an hour
- **Frozen vegetables** – Place a bag of these wrapped in a cloth against the affected area
- **Ginger** – Eat fresh, crystallised, in biscuits, or drink ginger tea
- **Horseradish** – Boil a cup of milk and mix in two tablespoons of grated horseradish. Soak a clean cloth in the mixture and apply to the affected area
- **Ice** – Apply ice wrapped in cloth to the affected area
- **Lavender** – Make a compress and apply to the affected areas
- **Lemon balm** – Soak a clean dressing in an infusion of lemon balm and apply to the affected joint as a warm, or cold, compress
- **Potato** – Boil chopped up new potatoes, strain, and soak cloth in broth and apply to affected joint
- **Turmeric** – Make a paste and apply to the affected area, fixing in place with cling film, or a dressing
- **Thyme** – Make thyme tea, allow to cool, soak a clean cloth in it, and apply to affected area for ten to fifteen minutes
- **Vinegar** – Rub warmed vinegar into the affected joint

Asthma

Asthma causes the lung airways to become inflamed, swollen, and narrowed, and causes excess mucus in the lungs. A number of things can trigger an attack of asthma including cough and cold infections, house dust mite dung, animal hair, stress, cold weather, and cigarette smoke. Some people with asthma get attacks when they exercise. The common symptoms are coughing, wheezing, and shortness of breath.

Conventional treatment

When triggers are identified it's important to avoid these. Generally there are two types of medication used – medication to relieve symptoms and medication to prevent symptoms from occurring.

Old-fashioned remedies

- **Apple** – Steam an apple, add two tablespoons of honey, mix together and consume. This helps to relieve a dry tickly cough and may help clear mucus

- **Brown sugar** – Added to a mixture of warm water and lemon juice to help soothe a tickly cough. Alternatively add it between layers of sliced raw onions in a bowl, and then use the resulting juice as a cough medicine
- **Liquorice** – To relieve an irritating and chesty cough mix powdered liquorice root with warm water, then gargle, and swallow

Athlete's foot

This is a very common and highly infectious fungal foot infection. Despite its name you don't have to be athletic to get it. The fungus is usually picked up from swimming pools or communal changing rooms and thrives in warm and moist parts of the body.

Athlete's foot begins as itchy, irritating patches of skin between the toes, which may peel, become soggy, crack, and even bleed. The fungus may infect the toenails and is often transported on underwear to the groins where it may cause "jock itch" fungal infection.

Conventional treatment

Keep feet and toes dry and use anti-fungal cream, spray, or powder as appropriate.

Old-fashioned remedies

- **Arnica** – Boil arnica flowers in water for five to ten minutes, strain the liquid and then apply to the athlete's foot using cotton wool once the liquid is at a temperature the skin can tolerate
- **Calendula** – Apply to the affected area as a cream or by soaking cotton wool in a cooled infusion
- **Garlic** – Crush a clove of garlic and rub against the affected area
- **Thyme** – Apply thyme tea tincture a few times a day. Alternatively make sufficient thyme tea to fill a bowl large enough to put both feet in, and rest the feet in the tea at as hot a temperature as can be tolerated
- **Yogurt** – Apply plain yogurt to the affected parts of the feet. Alternatively, if you have enough plain yogurt, soak the feet in a bowlful

Back pain

This is a very common problem that affects millions of people. It's usually the result of minor damage to the back muscles and ligaments caused when lifting or twisting, or sitting or standing in the wrong position. Being overweight also makes back pain more likely.

Back pain can come on suddenly or gradually and is usually felt around the lower back. It can make it difficult to get comfortable and to function normally. When a nerve in the back is irritated or pinched the pain travels to the buttocks and legs, called sciatica.

Conventional treatment

Painkillers are the mainstay of treatment for back pain. Exercise helps the back to recover so remaining as physically active as possible is best. It's no longer recommended to lie down for a long period of time. Heat packs, physiotherapy and massage therapy are helpful. Avoid further attacks of back pain by lifting correctly, losing excess weight, and keeping the back strong with exercise.

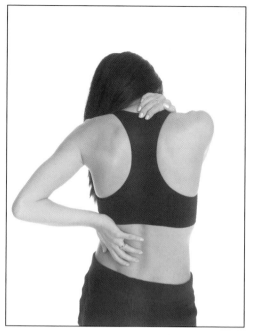

"Look after your back"

Old-fashioned remedies

- **Arnica** – Apply a warm poultice to the affected area
- **Basil** – Drink an infusion of basil
- **Bay leaf** – Soak in a hot bath with loose bay leaves added or tie leaves up in a small muslin cloth, soak in warm water, then rub gently against the sore area. Alternatively heat a handful of bay leaves in olive oil for fifteen to twenty minutes and then allow to simmer for a further ten minutes. Strain the oil, and rub against the affected area once cool enough to do so
- **Cabbage** – Place chilled cabbage leaves against the affected area and hold in place with a bandage. Alternatively warm up the leaves first, by blanching them in boiling water, running a hot iron over them, or putting them in a microwave. Place against sore area when temperature is tolerable, holding in place with a bandage
- **Horseradish** – Boil a cup of milk and mix in two tablespoons of grated horseradish. Soak a clean cloth in the mixture and apply to the affected area. The mixture, when cooled to a tolerable temperature, can also be massaged into the sore area
- **Rolling pin** – Massage the back with the rolling pin whilst standing with legs slightly apart, hold the rolling pin handles and roll it up and down the sore area

BAD BREATH

Bad breath, medically called halitosis, affects most people from time to time and often the person with bad breath isn't aware of it until it's pointed out to them. When this happens it can be very embarrassing and socially isolating. Poor oral hygiene is the number one cause of bad breath as this allows bacteria that live in the mouth to break down food particles releasing the smelly odours. Gum disease and tooth decay make bad breath more likely.

Smoking, stress, and not drinking enough liquid can make bad breath worse. Sometimes bad breath comes from a collection of bacteria at the back of the tongue.

Conventional treatment

Good dental hygiene by flossing and brushing each day usually prevents bad breath. Regular check-ups with the dentist helps identify and treat problems that left untreated contribute to bad breath. Not smoking and drinking more water can help, as can eating fewer odour-producing foods such as onions and garlic. Many benefit by using a tongue scraper to remove collections of bacteria from the back of the tongue.

Old-fashioned remedies

- **Cloves** – Chew one or two cloves and then spit these out
- **Lemon balm** – Drink lemon balm tea, warm or chilled
- **Liquorice** – Chew on liquorice root
- **Tomato** – Eat a tomato a few times a day as needed
- **Yogurt** – Eat a portion of yogurt each day

BLISTERS

Most blisters are filled with clear fluid called serum, and are caused by damage to the outer layer of the skin usually from heat as with burns, or friction and rubbing as with poorly fitting footwear. If a small blood vessel bursts a blood blister develops. If a blister becomes infected it may fill with pus.

Blisters can also form as the result of certain medical conditions such as chickenpox, herpes, and allergic reactions.

Conventional treatment

Don't burst the blister. It's there to protect the underlying skin whilst this heals. It will burst of its own accord and fluid will be reabsorbed naturally into the body. A plaster or clean dressing is used to cover the blister, particularly if it bursts before the skin has healed. Any underlying medical condition causing the blister can be treated as appropriate.

Old-fashioned remedies

- **Carrots** – Mash carrot and mix with a little olive oil or lard, apply to the blister and hold in place with a clean dressing
- **Honey** – Put honey onto a dressing and place over blister
- **Ice** – Apply to the blister in a clean cloth to relieve pain

Bloating

Bloating causes the abdomen to feel full, tight, and uncomfortable, and clothes to feel tight. There are many reasons for bloating including a high fibre diet, food intolerance, constipation, irritable bowel syndrome, premenstrual fluid retention, overeating, and air-swallowing due to anxiety, stress, and talking whilst eating too quickly. Less common, but more serious medical conditions associated with bloating include bowel obstruction, ascites, and tumours.

Conventional treatment

The first step is to identify what is causing bloating and to follow appropriate treatment advice. Medication can help disperse wind or treat causative conditions such as constipation. Increasing dietary fibre, more activity, taking time to eat in a relaxed manner, not eating on the go, and not talking whilst eating so less air is swallowed helps. Keeping stress under control is important.

Old-fashioned remedies

- **Basil** – Drink a cup of an infusion of basil after each meal
- **Ginger** – Eat grated fresh ginger, or crystallised ginger, or drink ginger tea after meals
- **Liquorice** – Chew and swallow liquorice, or take as powdered root with warm water, or as warm tea made from liquorice root
- **Peppermint** – Drink one or two cups of peppermint tea after each meal

High blood pressure

Medically known as hypertension high blood pressure damages the arteries that in turn may result in heart attack, stroke, kidney damage, and erectile dysfunction (impotence).

Invariably it doesn't cause symptoms, which is why it's a good idea to have it checked as regularly as advised by your doctor.

In most cases there's no specific cause but there's a greater risk of developing high blood pressure if it runs in the family and if someone is overweight, not very active, drinks too much alcohol, is stressed, and eats a high fat and high salt diet.

Conventional treatment

The first step is usually eliminating any risk factors by reducing salt consumption and eating a healthy diet, taking regular exercise, drinking less alcohol, losing weight if needed, and keeping stress under control. Medication to lower blood pressure is often needed.

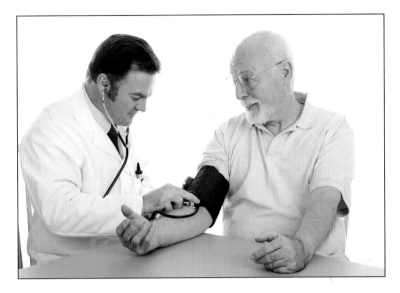

'Having your blood pressure taken is quick and painless'

Old-fashioned remedies

- **Bananas** – Eat one or two a day as they can help lower blood pressure
- **Cucumber** – Eat a quarter of a medium-sized cucumber each day
- **Garlic** – Consume three to four cloves a day. The allicin in garlic may help lower blood pressure
- **Ginger** – Use instead of salt to flavour dishes
- **Olive oil** – Consume one tablespoon each day
- **Omega-3** – Consume one to two portions of oily fish a week. Omega-3 essential fatty acids in these may help lower blood pressure

BODY ODOUR

Sweat is actually odourless but bacteria that normally live on the skin break down sweat into chemicals that smell, causing body odour that can be embarrassing and socially isolating for the person concerned. It's most often the armpits and genitals that smell because these parts of the body produce proteins and oily substances that bacteria feed on.

The smell is worse in hot and sweaty conditions, and can smell of foods eaten such as garlic and curry. Wearing unwashed clothes covered in sweat and bacteria will perpetuate body odour.

Conventional treatment

Regular baths and showers, washing the armpits and genital areas thoroughly, using deodorant or antiperspirant spray, and always wearing clean clothes will keep body odour away. Natural fibres such as cotton enable the skin to breathe so sweat evaporates more quickly. It can help to eat fewer hot and spicy foods.

Old-fashioned remedies

- **Bicarbonate of soda** – Dust some powder onto the skin of the armpits and genitals with a powder puff
- **Radish** – After bathing or showering pat the armpits and feet dry, and then apply a handful of radish juice under each armpit. Repeat this daily until the body odour no longer occurs
- **Vinegar** – Mix equal parts of apple cider vinegar and water then apply to the armpits daily, or to other parts of the body that are causing problems

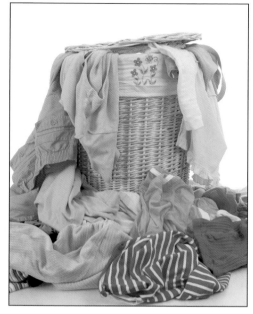

"Washing is the key to beating BO"

BREAST TENDERNESS

There are many reasons why breasts may feel uncomfortable, tender or painful. Hormone changes in the lead up to and during a period, or during pregnancy, are often responsible. When breastfeeding if milk is not emptied from the breast the milk ducts can become blocked causing mastitis when the breasts are swollen, red, sore and painful. Sometimes infection also develops as a consequence of the milk stagnating in the breast.

Conventional treatment

Rest, lots of liquid, paracetamol, and emptying the breasts of milk are the mainstay of treatment when breast-feeding. When infected, antibiotics are needed. When breasts are sore and painful, and a woman is not breast-feeding, anti-inflammatory medication can be used. Warmth on the breast can help as can wearing an appropriately fitted supportive bra.

Old-fashioned remedies

- **Arnica** – A cold compress of arnica or a warm poultice applied to the affected breast can help to reduce swelling, and ease soreness
- **Cabbage** – Place chilled cabbage against the affected breast by lining the bra cup with the leaves. Alternatively warm leaves up first by blanching them in boiling water, running a hot iron over them, or putting them in a microwave. Check that they are not too hot before using

- **Epsom salts** – Make a paste of Epsom salts with hot water and apply to the breast. Leave for ten to fifteen minutes and then wash off well
- **Frozen peas** – Wrap a bag of frozen vegetables in a soft cloth and place against the breast for five to ten minutes
- **Potato** – Make a potato poultice by boiling one or two large unpeeled potatoes until soft, then mash. Remove excess moisture and wrap in a cloth. Then place on the breast
- **Rolling pin** – Use to bruise the veins of cabbage leaves before applying these, warmed, to the sore breast

BRONCHITIS

This is an infection of the main lung airways, called the bronchi. It is often simply called a chest infection and when acute usually follows a cold or sore throat infection. Bronchitis causes a chesty hacking cough with mucus brought up, and sometimes wheezing and breathlessness. Some people have bronchitis all the time, called chronic bronchitis.

Conventional treatment

For most people bronchitis gets better on its own within a week – although the cough itself can last many weeks after this. Plenty of rest, liquid, and painkillers if necessary are usually all that's needed. Sometimes antibiotic treatment is necessary. Not smoking makes bronchitis less likely to develop. Some report improvements with supplements of vitamin C, zinc, and echinacea.

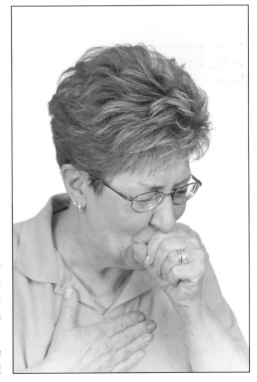

Old-fashioned remedies

- **Bay leaf** – Make a poultice of bay leaves after boiling these in water. When cool enough apply directly to the chest and cover with a dry cloth. Leave for up to thirty minutes
- **Lemon balm** – Lemon balm herbal tea can help reduce mucus production and ease irritating catarrh. Drinking a warm lemon balm herbal tea a couple of times a day can help
- **Liquorice** – Mix powdered liquorice root with warm water, then gargle, and swallow

"A cough is uncomfortable and disruptive"

BRUISES

Bruises appear when tiny blood vessels burst so blood leaks under the skin, usually as a consequence of an injury. Soon after the typical red or purple bruise appears it becomes green or yellow and then fades. When the bruise first appears it may feel uncomfortable.

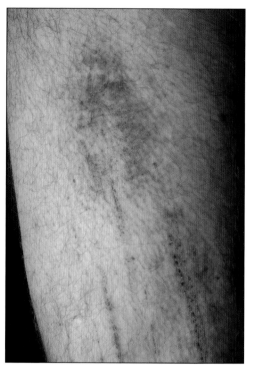

"Bruises appear when tiny blood vessels burst"

Conventional treatment

Painkillers and anti-inflammatory medication if the area is painful, but usually no specific treatment is needed other than some tender loving care.

Old-fashioned remedies

- **Arnica** – Put a few drops of arnica tincture onto a clean cloth or dressing to make a compress and apply to the bruised area of the body
- **Banana** – Apply the inside of the peel against the bruise, bandage this in place, and leave for twelve to twenty-four hours
- **Brown sugar** – Immediately a bruise begins to appear spread molasses on brown paper and apply to the bruise
- **Epsom salts** – Add a few tablespoons of Epsom salts to warm bath water and relax. Alternatively, make a paste of Epsom salts with hot water and apply to the bruised area. Leave for ten to fifteen minutes and then wash off well
- **Frozen vegetables** – Wrap in a cloth and apply to the bruised area for up to five minutes
- **Ice** – Wrap ice cubes in a cloth and apply to the bruised area for up to five minutes
- **Onions** – Place a poultice of grated onion and salt against the bruise
- **Peppermint** – Allow a cup of peppermint tea to cool and then soak a clean cloth with this. Press against the affected area and hold in place with a bandage
- **Potato** – Apply grated potato to the bruised area
- **Radish** – Grate a daikon radish and apply the gratings directly to the bruised area. Keep in place for twenty to thirty minutes with a clean dressing. Continue this once or twice a day as needed. Radish juice can also be used for this complaint
- **Vinegar** – Apply cooled vinegar to the bruised area with a compress for ten to twenty minutes. Repeat this a few times during the day
- **Witch hazel** – Apply witch hazel to the bruised part using tea, tincture, or a cream

BURNS

Burns are caused by direct contact with heat or a flame, scalds by liquid or steam. Both can be very painful. Most often they are superficial with skin becoming red, a little swollen, and painful.

Conventional treatment

Burns and scalds need treatment as soon as possible to minimise the potential damage to the skin. Run the area under cool water for at least ten minutes to cool it, relieve pain, and reduce the risk of infection. Cover it with cling film or a clean dressing. Painkillers and anti-inflammatory drugs are used to relieve pain. Any burn or scald larger than a postage stamp should receive medical attention. Medicated creams can be used to prevent or treat any infection.

Old-fashioned remedies

- **Aloe vera** – Apply to the burned area
- **Brown sugar** – Ensure the wound is clean then sprinkle the wound lightly with brown sugar, holding in place with petroleum jelly around the wound and protecting with a clean dressing. Repeat this process once or twice daily
- **Calendula** – Apply as a poultice, compress, cream or ointment
- **Carrots** – Soak a clean dressing in carrot juice and apply to the affected area
- **Honey** – Apply a thin coating of honey, and cover with a clean dressing
- **Lavender** – Make a lavender infusion using the flowers, strain and leave until the temperature is tolerable to the skin. Apply directly to the affected area or as a compress
- **Onions** – Cut a raw onion in half and rub against the burn
- **Papaya** – Place a slice of papaya pulp over the burn and keep this in place with a sterile bandage or sticking plaster
- **Radish** – Mix mashed radish with crushed ice until a consistency thick enough to apply to the scald or burn. Cover with a clean dressing or cling film and leave for ten to fifteen minutes. Radish juice can also be used for this complaint
- **Thyme** – Apply cooled thyme tea directly to the affected area or by using a clean cloth soaked in the tea. Thyme tea can also be applied to a clean dressing, which is then applied to the affected area

WARNING:
It's important to run the burn under cool water first, and then allow twenty to thirty minutes before applying any of the old-fashioned remedies described above.

CHAPPED LIPS

Lips become chapped and sore from time to time, often the result of exposure to cold dry air, sun, or wind. Dehydration makes the lips feel dry and can cause chapping, as can the habit of lip-licking. If the lips come into contact with something that irritates them such as a cosmetic or lip-care product these may cause chapped lips too.

Conventional treatment

It's important to protect the lips with a lip balm or lubricating cream, which ideally contains UV protection. Petroleum jelly has traditionally been used by many people to protect the lips from exposure to the environment. Also, keeping hydrated and not licking the lips, whilst avoiding any known irritants is important.

Old-fashioned remedies

- **Cranberry** – Take a dozen cranberries and microwave these for a couple of minutes. Mash these, allow to cool, strain, and store in a jar or other suitable container. Apply to the chapped lips
- **Ice** – Apply ice wrapped in cloth to the affected area
- **Lemon balm** – Chop up a few leaves and mix with yogurt until the consistency of a cream and apply to the affected area. Cooling in the fridge can make it more effective. Alternatively soak a lemon balm tea bag in hot water for three to five minutes and once at a tolerable temperature apply it to the affected area
- **Tea** – Soak a tea bag in warm water and press against lips for two to three minutes. Alternatively place a soaked tea bag in the refrigerator to cool and then apply to lips

CHICKENPOX

This infection is very contagious and is caused by the varicella-zoster virus. It's characterised by a rash that begins as small, itchy red spots, that become extremely itchy fluid-filled blisters, that in turn crust over forming scabs that after a week or two will fall off. Don't pick these as doing so makes secondary infection and scarring more likely. This virus lies dormant in the body and may later be reactivated causing shingles.

Conventional treatment

Although there's no specific treatment for chickenpox applying calamine lotion to the spots helps relieve itching and paracetamol reduces any fever and relieves any discomfort or pain. Sometimes antiviral medicine is recommended.

Old-fashioned remedies

- **Bicarbonate of soda** – Apply a solution of bicarbonate of soda and water, or mix bicarbonate of soda with olive oil, to the itchy part of the body
- **Carrots** – Apply freshly cut slices of carrot to the itchy areas. Cooled slices may bring even greater relief
- **Milk** – Add a tablespoon of salt to a cup of milk, mix together then apply to the area affected. Leave to dry on the skin
- **Oatmeal** – Make an oatmeal paste by mixing uncooked oatmeal and water, and apply to the itchy areas either directly or by placing in muslin cloth. Add oatmeal to the bath by wrapping two handfuls of oatmeal in muslin, tying to make a bag, and dropping in the water
- **Olive oil** – Mix olive oil with bicarbonate of soda and apply to itchy areas
- **Turmeric** – Mix together coconut oil with turmeric powder and gently apply to the affected area
- **Vinegar** – Mix two tablespoons of vinegar with a cup of water and apply to the affected area
- **Witch hazel** – Soak a cotton wool ball or a clean cloth in witch hazel tea and apply to the affected area

CHILBLAINS

An abnormal skin reaction to cold causes small, itchy, and often painful red swellings to appear, usually on the toes, fingers, ear lobes and the tip of the nose where the skin is cooler.

Conventional treatment

Keeping warm, and exercising before going out in cold weather, may help to improve blood flow to the extremities. Medication may be recommended to prevent chilblains when they keep on recurring. Creams can help to relieve itching and soreness whilst the body naturally heals the chilblain.

Old-fashioned remedies

- **Oatmeal** – Make an oatmeal paste by mixing uncooked oatmeal and water, and apply to the itchy areas either directly or by placing in muslin cloth
- **Onion** – Soak the feet in warm water and then rub the dried feet with sliced raw onion
- **Salt** – Rub brandy and salt over the affected area. Alternatively, mix a few handfuls of salt in hot water, and when at a comfortable temperature bathe the feet or hands
- **Tea** – Steep four tea bags in boiling water for ten minutes. Allow to cool, and then apply liquid to affected area using a cloth

- **Yogurt** – Apply directly to the skin, allow to dry and leave for ten to fifteen minutes, before rinsing off with cool water

COLD SORES

Cold sores are caused by an infection with the herpes simplex virus and are very contagious so are easily contracted through close contact with someone who gets cold sores. First of all there's usually a tingling sensation that's soon followed by a blister-like sore somewhere around the mouth. This can be itchy, painful, and embarrassing.

Conventional treatment.

Antiviral cream may help to nip an attack in the bud or make an attack shorter and painkillers relieve pain and discomfort.

Repeat attacks can be triggered by emotional upset, cough and cold infections, menstrual periods, fatigue, cold winds and UV exposure from bright sunlight so these are best avoided. A UV protection lip balm can help make further attacks less likely.

Old-fashioned remedies

- **Aloe vera** – Rub fresh gel against the cold sore a couple of times a day
- **Calendula** – Can be applied as a tincture, poultice, compress, cream or ointment. Doing this as soon as the tell tale tingling starts may stop a cold sore in its tracks
- **Garlic** – Crush a clove of garlic and rub against the cold sore. Doing this as soon as the tell-tale tingling starts may stop a cold sore in its tracks
- **Ice** – Apply an ice cube to the cold sore. Doing this as soon as the tell tale tingling starts may stop a cold sore in its tracks
- **Lemon balm** – After allowing a lemon balm herbal teabag to cool apply to the sore. Alternatively lemon balm can be applied as a cream. Doing this as soon as the tell tale tingling starts may stop a cold sore in its tracks
- **Witch hazel** – Apply witch hazel daily to the cold sore

CONSTIPATION

Constipation can mean not opening the bowels at all but it is also when someone has to strain more than usual, is not going as often as usual, and doesn't feel that they are emptying their bowels completely. Often the bowel motions are hard, lumpy, small like rabbit-pellets, or very large.

When someone is constipated they may experience bloating, excess wind, nausea, abdominal discomfort and cramps, a lack of energy and a loss of appetite. People who are constipated often feel full up quickly when eating.

Not eating enough fibre or drinking enough liquid, inactivity, stress, and ignoring the call of Nature make constipation more likely, as does pregnancy and some medical conditions such as irritable bowel syndrome (IBS).

Conventional treatment

Consuming more fibre and fluid in the diet, exercise, reducing stress, and responding to Nature's call helps treat, and prevent, constipation. When necessary laxatives and bulk-forming agents are used to get things moving again.

Old-fashioned remedies

- **Aloe vera** – Take aloe vera juice as directed on the product packaging
- **Bananas** – Eat one or two a day
- **Brown sugar** – Drink a solution of one to two teaspoons of brown sugar in warm water

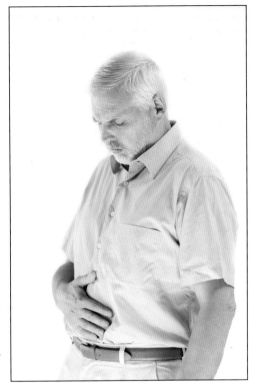

"Constipation often causes bloating and stomach ache"

- **Cabbage** – Eat three to four cooked leaves each day
- **Cucumber** – Consume one quarter of a medium-sized cucumber and repeat daily as required
- **Epsom salts** – Follow the dosage directions on the packet. If this is not possible dissolve a teaspoon of Epsom salts in a cup of warm water and drink
- **Liquorice** – Chew and swallow liquorice or mix half a teaspoon of liquorice root powder with warm water and drink. Liquorice tea can also be used
- **Oats** – Eat a bowl of porridge or muesli each morning
- **Olive oil** – Take one teaspoon twice a day and increase as needed
- **Papaya** – Eat ripe fruit or make the fruit into juice and drink

CORNS AND CALLUSES

Corns are small areas of very thick skin, that may be hard, occurring on top or on the outside of toes, or soft, occurring between the toes where the natural moisture of sweat keeps them soft. Calluses are larger areas of hard skin that usually appear on the sole. Pressure on the skin, or rubbing because of poorly fitting footwear for instance, causes corns and calluses that may simply be unsightly but can become painful.

Conventional treatment

Removing hard skin can be done with a pumice stone or emery board and moisturising the feet each day helps. Medicated solutions and corn plasters are best used under the supervision of a podiatrist. For soft corns keeping in between the toes dry with a drying powder helps. Wearing comfortable and properly fitting footwear will lessen the chance of corns and calluses developing or returning.

Old-fashioned remedies

- **Cranberry** – Mash one or two handfuls of fresh cranberries and using a bandage secure these over the corn or callus. Leave for twenty to thirty minutes. Repeat daily as required
- **Lemon juice** – Place a slice of lemon over the corn and keep it in place with tape and leave overnight. Repeat this daily until corn has gone
- **Oats** – Add a cup of oatmeal to a litre of boiling water and continue boiling until water has reduced by around twenty-five per cent volume. Strain this and soak feet in the water once cool enough to tolerate. Remove oatmeal from the strainer and use to exfoliate the feet whilst they are soaking
- **Onions** – Mash roasted onions with soap and apply to the feet in a poultice
- **Papaya** – Drip the milky latex from a green papaya onto the corn or callus two to three times daily until gone
- **Peppermint** – Add to natural yogurt and massage into the corn or callus, or soak the feet for around thirty minutes in a bowl filled with warm peppermint tea, or warm water with half a dozen drops of peppermint oil added
- **Tea** – Moisten a tea bag and then tape against the corn or callus. Leave in place for thirty to sixty minutes
- **Vinegar** – Soften by soaking the feet in a footbath of warm water and vinegar for twenty to thirty minutes

Coughs and colds

Adults can get up to five of these infections a year, which are caused by more than two hundred different viruses. Common symptoms include a sore throat, runny and blocked nose, sneezing, and a cough.

Conventional treatment

Antibiotics do not help to treat the common cold as they treat only those infections caused by bacteria, not viruses. Rest, drinking plenty of fluid, and painkiller and decongestant medication relieve symptoms. Some recommend taking high doses of vitamin C, additional zinc, the herb echinacea, or pelargonium to try and shorten the duration and severity of the infection.

Old-fashioned remedies

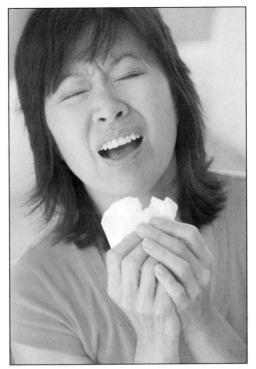

- **Apple** – Steam an apple, add two tablespoons of honey, mix together and consume. This helps to relieve a dry tickly cough and may help clear mucus
- **Basil** – Make a decoction of basil leaves by mashing the leaves and then boiling these in water. Ginger and honey can be added if desired. Allow to cool and then drink
- **Brown sugar** – Brown sugar can be added to a mixture of warm water and lemon juice to help soothe a tickly cough and sore throat. Another way of making use of brown sugar is to add it between layers of sliced raw onions in a bowl, and then use the resulting juice as a cough medicine

"Cough and sneeze into a disposable tissue to prevent spreading infection"

- **Garlic** – Eat up to three cloves a day
- **Ginger** – Finely grate fresh ginger into a cup and add boiling water. Allow to sit until at a comfortable temperature then gargle and swallow. Do this as needed. A spoonful of honey and a squeeze of lemon juice can be added if desired
- **Honey** – A spoonful of honey alone will do the trick. Alternatively to warm water add a spoonful of honey and a squeeze of lemon juice and mix these together. This can be gargled and then swallowed as needed
- **Horseradish** – Relieve nasal congestion and clear mucus from the chest by slicing horseradish root and breathing in deeply. Chew slices of horseradish starting with a small slice and increase the amount as needed
- **Liquorice** – Mix powdered liquorice root with warm water, then gargle, and swallow
- **Peppermint** – Inhale the steam of hot water with peppermint oil added, taking care not to get too close to avoid the nasal passages getting burned
- **Thyme** – Allow thyme tea to cool to a temperature that can be tolerated then gargle the liquid. Do this as often as needed
- **Tonic water** – Drink a glass for the possible anti-inflammatory, painkilling, and fever-reducing effects of quinine. Add some lemon if desired

CRADLE CAP

Cradle cap occurs in babies when dead skin cells and excess sebum – the oil produced by glands in the skin to prevent skin and hair drying out – clog the skin pores. It's medically known as seborrhoeic dermatitis, and is not infectious or caused by poor hygiene. It usually clears by the time a baby reaches his first birthday and is harmless to a baby but often causes parents distress because of its appearance.

Conventional treatment

The scales can be loosened by rubbing olive oil into the scalp, leaving it overnight, and washing it off the following day using an ordinary baby shampoo or a cream. The scales should not be picked as this may damage the scalp. If it becomes infected antibiotic or anti-fungal treatment may be used, and if it becomes inflamed steroid cream may be recommended.

Old-fashioned remedies

- **Olive oil** – The scales can be loosened by rubbing olive oil into the scalp, leaving it overnight, and washing it off the following day using an ordinary baby shampoo or a cream

CROUP

This infection of the larynx and the windpipe (trachea) that's commonest in winter usually affects young children and causes a 'seal-like' barking cough. Children often have a fever, runny nose, a hoarse voice, and the infection can make breathing difficult.

Conventional treatment

There's no specific treatment as the body fights the infection. Tender loving care is important as a child is easily frightened by this infection. Medicine to treat fever and any discomfort is often recommended, as is plenty of liquid to combat any dehydration. Sometimes treatment in hospital is needed to help a child breathe more easily.

Old-fashioned remedies

- **Steam** – Sit in a bathroom with the hot taps running so the room is filled with steam

CUTS AND GRAZES

Children fall down, and adults cut themselves preparing vegetables in the kitchen, doing DIY, shaving, or just opening an envelope. Usually bleeding is minor and the cut or graze feels sore. Scabs often form as part of the healing process and sometimes a scar is left as a gentle reminder. Sometimes the wound becomes infected.

Conventional treatment

Wash hands thoroughly, clean the wound under running water, and pat dry with a clean towel. Bleeding can be stopped by applying firm pressure to the wound. Once bleeding has stopped apply a plaster or sterile dressing and keep clean. For painful cuts, grazes, or wounds painkillers can help. If the wound becomes infected antibiotics may be needed. If the bleeding will not stop seek medical advice.

Old fashioned remedies

- **Brown sugar** – A good antiseptic. Ensure wound is clean then sprinkle the wound lightly with brown sugar. Smear petroleum jelly around the wound to hold the grains of sugar in place and then protect with a clean dressing
- **Frozen vegetables** – Wrap a bag of frozen vegetables in a soft cloth and apply to the affected area
- **Ice** – Wrap ice cubes in a soft cloth, and apply to the affected area
- **Honey** – A good antiseptic. After cleaning the wound with water and patting it dry apply honey to a clean dressing and place the honey coated side of the dressing against the wound
- **Lavender** – A good antiseptic. Make a lavender infusion using the flowers, strain and leave until the temperature is at a level tolerable to the skin. Apply directly to the affected area or as a compress
- **Lemon juice** – Drip lemon juice onto the cut to stop bleeding
- **Turmeric** – Ensure the wound is clean then sprinkle turmeric powder onto it to stop bleeding and cover with a clean dressing
- **Witch hazel** – Apply a few drops of witch hazel tincture to the cut using a cotton bud to stop bleeding

CYSTITIS

Irritation, damage or most often infection causes inflammation of the bladder lining, called cystitis. It's much more common for women to be affected but men can be too. Burning, stinging or pain when passing urine, and needing to go more than usual but only passing small quantities of urine are the usual symptoms.

Conventional treatment

Drinking plenty of water, taking painkillers, and using sachets of sodium citrate or potassium citrate to neutralise any acidity relieves symptoms of cystitis that often resolves in a matter of days. Sometimes a course of antibiotics is recommended.

Old-fashioned remedies

- **Bicarbonate of soda** – Drink half a teaspoon of bicarbonate of soda dissolved in water
- **Cranberry** – Drink 250mls of cranberry juice in the morning, and another of the same in the evening
- **Salt** – Add a tablespoon of salt to a bath of warm water, climb in and relax

DANDRUFF

It's normal for old skin cells on the scalp to fall off, but if these clump together then dandruff occurs, usually being obvious either in the hair or on clothing. A fungal infection often causes dandruff, and salty, sugary, and spicy diets and too much alcohol can make things worse, as can stress.

Conventional treatment

An antidandruff shampoo is what most people try first, making sure to wash the hair every day, thoroughly rinsing it, and not using hair care products or heat drying if these dry the scalp. Anti-fungal or tea tree shampoo is often recommended. Reducing consumption of alcohol, sugar, salty and spicy foods for a while can help, as can managing stress.

Old-fashioned remedies

- **Bay leaf** – Crumble half a dozen bay leaves and add these to boiling water. Allow to brew for thirty minutes, strain and put into a container to cool. Rinse hair with water, massage the bay tea into the hair, wait a few minutes and repeat with more bay tea. Leave for about one hour then rinse out
- **Coconut oil** – Massage coconut oil into the scalp, and leave overnight. The following morning rinse hair. Repeat this nightly as required to keep dandruff at bay
- **Lemon juice** – Mix the juice of half a lemon into two cups of water, apply the juice from the other half of the lemon to the hair. Wash hair with shampoo first, then rinse with water, and then with the lemon and water mixture already prepared. Repeat this daily until dandruff has cleared
- **Vinegar** – Soak the scalp and hair with vinegar, leaving for an hour or so, and then rinse

"Nothing feels good with depression"

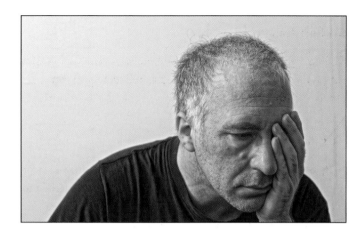

DEPRESSION

Depression makes people feel low and lacking interest or pleasure in the things they would normally enjoy. It lasts for a long time, more than a couple of weeks, and can also detrimentally affect sleep patterns, appetite, ability to concentrate, and mood. It's often, but not always, triggered by a life event such as bereavement, job loss, or the break-up of a relationship. An imbalance of chemical hormones in the body may cause depression too as may a change in social circumstances. There are specific types of depression such as seasonal affective disorder that most often occurs during the winter months, and post-natal depression.

Conventional treatment

Exercise, the herb St John's Wort, counselling, and antidepressants are all options for treating depression. Which is used depends upon the individual's preference and the severity of the depression.

Old-fashioned remedies

- **Lemon balm** – Drink a warm lemon balm tea a couple of times a day
- **Onions** – Eat half an onion each day

DIARRHOEA

When it's short-term diarrhoea, passing watery stools frequently, is usually caused by infection, food poisoning, or something consumed that was too spicy or the body isn't used to. Diarrhoea can be more long-term, a consequence of conditions such as irritable bowel syndrome, lactose intolerance, Crohn's disease, ulcerative colitis, and anxiety. Medication side effects can be responsible too.

Conventional treatment

Avoiding dehydration is the most important measure by drinking plenty of liquid or using rehydration drinks. In fact, medical advice nowadays is to continue eating as normally as possible. Anti-diarrhoea medication can also be used. Some find that eating more fibre helps to bind the motions.

Old-fashioned remedies

- **Apple** – Grate a raw unpeeled apple, place on a plate or in a dish for fifteen to twenty minutes until it turns brown and oxidised. Then eat the browned apple, which can be mixed with banana if desired
- **Bananas** – Eat one or two each day as needed
- **Brown sugar** – Drink a solution of one to two teaspoons of brown sugar in warm water
- **Cloves** – Add a few drops of clove oil to water and drink

DRY SKIN

Most people get dry skin over parts of the body from time to time. This may itch, be flaky, feel a little uncomfortable, or may make them feel self-conscious because of its appearance. Exposure to sun, wind, or cold air; irritation from clothing or skin-care products; dehydration; and stress are often responsible for the skin becoming dry and chapped. Long-term skin conditions such as eczema and psoriasis cause dry skin too.

Conventional treatment

The usual treatment is to keep the skin well moisturised, keep the body hydrated, whilst avoiding any identified causes of skin dryness.

Old-fashioned remedies

- **Aloe vera** – Apply fresh gel to the affected area and gently rub in
- **Apples** – Cut an apple in half and then rub it against the skin
- **Calendula** – Apply as a tincture, poultice, compress, cream or ointment
- **Bicarbonate of soda** – Mix bicarbonate of soda and water and apply to affected area
- **Carrots** – Apply freshly cut slices of carrot to the itchy areas
- **Coconut oil** – Apply to the affected area. Turmeric can be mixed with the coconut oil if desired
- **Cucumber** – Place a slice of cucumber against the sore skin or grind cucumber into a paste and then apply to sore area of skin
- **Frozen vegetables** – Place a bag of these wrapped in a cloth against the affected area

- **Horseradish** – Juice slices of horseradish and add to honey then apply to the affected areas
- **Ice** – Apply ice wrapped in cloth to the affected area
- **Oatmeal** – Make an oatmeal paste by mixing uncooked oatmeal and water, and apply to the itchy areas either directly or by placing in muslin cloth
- **Olive oil** – Pour some into the palm of the hand and gently massage into the skin
- **Milk** – Add a tablespoon of salt to a cup of milk, mix together, then apply to affected area, and leave to dry
- **Potato** – Rub the flesh of half a potato against affected area or grate a potato and apply as a poultice
- **Tea** – Steep four tea bags in boiling water for ten minutes. Allow to cool, and then apply liquid to affected area using a cloth
- **Tomato** – Puree peeled tomatoes and add to a spoonful of yogurt or a spoonful of buttermilk and then apply. Alternatively slice the tomatoes, dip in yogurt or buttermilk and apply to affected areas
- **Turmeric** – Mix together coconut oil with turmeric powder and gently apply to the affected area
- **Vinegar** – Mix two tablespoons of vinegar with a cup of water and apply to affected area
- **Witch hazel** – Apply to the skin with a cotton wool ball or clean cloth soaked in witch hazel tea
- **Yogurt** – Apply directly to the skin, allow to dry and leave for ten to fifteen minutes, before rinsing off with cool water

Eczema

This condition causes the skin to become dry, red, itchy, and cracked, and is also known as dermatitis. The commonest type of eczema is atopic eczema and is very common in children, but adults can be affected too. Those with allergies are more prone to developing this type of eczema. Often flare-ups are triggered by exposure to house dust mite dung, pet hairs, certain foods, infection, and stress.

Other types of eczema that cause similar skin problems are seborrhoeic eczema when too much sebum, the oily liquid that stops the hair and skin drying out, is produced by the sebaceous glands in the skin, and contact eczema where symptoms are triggered by contact with an irritant substance, for example a hair-care product, or with a substance that a person is allergic to such as nickel.

Conventional treatment

Eczema is treated with regular moisturising, steroid creams and ointments, and other treatments applied to the skin. Sometimes antibiotics are also used when the eczema becomes infected. Those things that trigger flare-ups are best avoided.

Old-fashioned remedies

- **Aloe vera** – Apply fresh gel to the affected area and gently rub in
- **Apples** – Cut an apple in half and then rub it against the skin
- **Bicarbonate of soda** – Mix bicarbonate of soda and water and apply to affected area
- **Calendula** – Apply as a tincture, poultice, compress, cream or ointment
- **Carrots** – Apply freshly cut slices of carrot to the itchy areas
- **Coconut oil** – Apply to the affected area. Turmeric can be mixed with the coconut oil if desired
- **Cucumber** – Place a slice of cucumber against the sore skin or grind cucumber into a paste and then apply to sore area of skin
- **Frozen vegetables** – Place a bag of these wrapped in a cloth against the affected area
- **Horseradish** – Juice slices of horseradish and add to honey then apply to the affected areas
- **Ice** – Apply ice wrapped in cloth to the affected area
- **Oatmeal** – Make an oatmeal paste by mixing uncooked oatmeal and water, and apply to the itchy areas either directly or by placing in muslin cloth
- **Olive oil** – Pour some into the palm of the hand and gently massage into the skin
- **Milk** – Add a tablespoon of salt to a cup of milk, mix together, then apply to affected area, and leave to dry
- **Potato** – Rub the flesh of half a potato against affected area or grate a potato and apply as a poultice
- **Tea** – Steep four tea bags in boiling water for ten minutes. Allow to cool, and then apply liquid to affected area using a cloth
- **Tomato** – Puree peeled tomatoes and add to a spoonful of yogurt or a spoonful of buttermilk and then apply. Alternatively slice the tomatoes, dip in yogurt or buttermilk and apply to affected areas
- **Turmeric** – Mix together coconut oil with turmeric powder and gently apply to the affected area
- **Vinegar** – Mix two tablespoons of vinegar with a cup of water and apply to affected area
- **Witch hazel** – Apply to the skin with a cotton wool ball or clean cloth soaked in witch hazel tea
- **Yogurt** – Apply directly to the skin, allow to dry and leave for ten to fifteen minutes, before rinsing off with cool water

EYE BAGS

Dark bags under the eyes are often caused by being overtired. A lack of sleep or simply doing too much in the day may be responsible. Sometimes it's due to a person's cultural skin tones.

Conventional treatment

Getting enough rest, relaxation and sleep is a good start. Eating healthily, drinking enough water, not smoking, and drinking safe amounts of alcohol helps the skin to look good. Some people use cover-up make-up.

Old-fashioned remedies

- **Camomile** – Brew a cup of camomile tea, remove the tea bag and allow to cool until it's at a temperature that can be tolerated and rest it against closed eyes
- **Cucumber** – Place a chilled slice of cucumber over the closed eyelids
- **Papaya** – Make a poultice of mashed papaya fruit and place over closed eyes
- **Potato** – Extract juice from one or two potatoes, soak cotton wool in the juice, and gently hold against closed eyes
- **Tea** – Add a tea bag to boiled water, leave for around five minutes and then remove, squeeze out and allow to cool to a tolerable temperature then place over closed eyes
- **Thyme** – Make a compress of thyme tea and place gently over closed eyes

FEVER

When a person's body temperature rises above normal they are said to have a fever. Medically speaking a temperature above thirty-eight degrees centigrade is considered a significant fever and occurs because of the release of chemicals by the immune system in response to infection and inflammation. Infections are the main culprits for fever, but hot weather and inflammatory conditions such as rheumatoid arthritis can also be responsible.

Conventional treatment

Paracetamol or ibuprofen both lower temperature. Keeping hydrated helps to reduce temperature as does being in a cool environment and wearing minimal clothing.

Old-fashioned remedies

- **Feverfew** – Make an infusion of the dried leaves and drink this
- **Ice** – Suck and roll ice cubes around the mouth
- **Thyme** – Make a thyme tea compress and place against the forehead
- **Tonic water** – Drink a glass of tonic water

FOOT PROBLEMS

From time to time most people experience tired, sore, or aching feet. It may be because of being on the feet all day, or because shoes that win fashion awards deserve no award for the discomfort they inflict on the feet. Arthritis, hard skin, verrucas, and other health complaints can cause problems with the feet.

Conventional treatment

Resting the feet and keeping them up when possible literally takes the pressure off feet. Bathing them in warm water is very soothing and relaxing, as is giving them, or allowing them to be massaged. Treating any foot problems such as athlete's foot, verrucas, corns and calluses, and joint deformities such as bunions makes foot problems less likely.

Old-fashioned remedies

- **Epsom salts** – Mix a pinch of Epsom salts with olive oil and rub onto the skin to relieve aching, washing off after around five to ten minutes
- **Horseradish** – Take one or two horseradish leaves and gently blanch these. Remove any fibres running through the leaves and then strap to the bottom of the feet with a bandage. Leave for around thirty minutes to relieve aching
- **Oats** – Make an oatmeal paste by mixing uncooked oatmeal and water, and apply to the feet either directly or by placing in muslin cloth to relieve dryness
- **Peppermint** – Add peppermint oil to yogurt and massage into the feet to relieve aching. Alternatively soak the feet for around thirty minutes in a bowl filled with warm peppermint tea, or warm water with half a dozen drops of peppermint oil added
- **Rolling pin** – Soak feet in warm water for ten to fifteen minutes. Dry thoroughly. Whilst sitting place each foot in turn on the rolling pin, or together if the pin is long enough, and roll the pin forwards and backwards using the feet to relieve aching
- **Thyme** – Make thyme tea, allow to cool, and soak feet in this for ten to fifteen minutes to relieve aching
- **Tomato** – Ease aching feet by wrapping slices of tomatoes on the soles of the feet for twenty to thirty minutes. Alternatively place sliced tomatoes in an oval baking dish long enough to place feet in. Sit with feet resting on tomato slices for twenty to thirty minutes. If necessary use two dishes, one for each foot
- **Yogurt** – Apply directly to the skin, allow to dry and leave for ten to fifteen minutes before rinsing off with cool water to relieve dryness

GOUT

Gout is a form of arthritis caused by excess uric acid in the blood which can form needle-like crystals that attack the joints causing excruciating pain, swelling and inflammation. Attacks of gout are triggered by stress, injury, being overweight, some medication, and foods, for example liver, kidneys, and herring, and alcohol such as beer, that are high in purines, the chemicals which increase levels of uric acid in the blood. Any joint can be affected but in most cases the first one is the big toe.

Conventional treatment

During an attack of gout rest, ice, painkillers and anti-inflammatory medication are available to relieve swelling and pain. To prevent further attacks preventative medication may be recommended to reduce the amount of urate in the blood. Losing weight if needed, and avoiding foods and drinks that trigger attacks is sensible.

Old-fashioned remedies

- **Arnica** – Apply a tincture of arnica to the affected joint or joints with a compress or poultice and fix to the joint with a bandage and leave for fifteen to twenty minutes
- **Bay leaf** – Tie leaves up in a small muslin cloth and soak in hot water, allow to cool, and then gently rub against the sore area. Alternatively, heat a handful of bay leaves in olive oil for fifteen to twenty minutes, allow to simmer for a further ten minutes, strain the oil, and rub against the affected area once cool enough to do so
- **Basil** – Drink an infusion of basil twice a day
- **Cabbage** – Place chilled cabbage leaves against the affected joint and leave for a couple of hours. Alternatively, warm up the leaves first by blanching in boiling water, running a hot iron over them, or putting them in a microwave
- **Feverfew** – Soak a clean cloth in a freshly brewed feverfew infusion and apply to the affected joint. If more than one joint is affected it may be simpler to consume a cup of weak feverfew tea
- **Figs** – Soak four figs in water and then mash these into a poultice. Apply directly to the affected area and keep in place with a clean cloth or dressing. Leave for thirty minutes to an hour
- **Frozen vegetables** – Place a bag of these wrapped in a cloth against the affected area
- **Horseradish** – Boil a cup of milk and mix in two tablespoons of grated horseradish. Soak a clean cloth in the mixture and apply to the affected area
- **Ice** – Apply ice wrapped in cloth to the affected area
- **Lavender** – Make a compress and apply to the affected area
- **Lemon balm** – Soak a clean dressing in an infusion of lemon balm and apply to the affected joint as a warm, or cold, compress
- **Potato** – Boil chopped up new potatoes, strain, and soak cloth in broth and apply to affected joint
- **Thyme** – Make thyme tea, allow to cool, soak a clean cloth in it, and apply to affected area
- **Turmeric** – Make a paste and apply to the affected area, fixing in place with cling film, or a dressing
- **Vinegar** – Rub warmed vinegar into the affected joint

HAEMORRHOIDS

Haemorrhoids, or piles as they're commonly known, occur when pressure – usually from straining on the toilet or a pregnant tummy – causes blood vessels lining the back passage to swell, rather like varicose veins.

Pregnancy, natural childbirth, and constipation are common causes of haemorrhoids, which can bleed, feel uncomfortable or itchy, or be felt as a lump around the back passage.

"Cheerful relief"

Conventional treatment

Haemorrhoids are usually treated with cream, ointment, spray, or suppositories. Eating plenty of fibre, drinking plenty of liquid, and responding to Nature's call helps avoid constipation and straining and consequently haemorrhoids. Sometimes an operation is needed to remove the haemorrhoids.

Old-fashioned remedies

- **Aloe vera** – Apply to the affected part after opening the bowels and wiping the area
- **Arnica** – Apply a cold compress or a warm poultice to the affected area
- **Calendula** – Apply as cream or ointment, or make an infusion of calendula leaves and having soaked a clean cloth with this, apply to the affected area. It can be applied as a warm poultice too
- **Cloves** – Mix clove oil with yogurt and apply as a cream
- **Cranberry** – Blend a cup of cranberries then wrap a tablespoonful in muslin and place against the haemorrhoids for thirty minutes
- **Frozen vegetables** – Sit on a bag of frozen vegetables wrapped in a cloth
- **Ice** – Sit on a bag of ice wrapped in a clean cloth
- **Onions** – Slice a raw onion and mix with one to two teaspoons of honey. Put in a fresh dressing and apply to the haemorrhoids for a few hours
- **Potato** – Apply grated potato to the swollen area
- **Turmeric** – Make a paste by mixing two tablespoons of turmeric into boiling water. Add one tablespoon of lemon or lime juice if desired. Apply paste to haemorrhoids and hold in place for twenty to thirty minutes with a clean cloth by taping if possible. If not, sit on it

- **Witch hazel** – Soak a clean cloth in witch hazel tea and apply to the haemorrhoids two or three times a day for five to ten minutes. Alternatively apply a few drops of witch hazel tincture to the haemorrhoids using a cotton bud

HANGOVER

We pay the price for drinking too much alcohol with a hangover. Chemicals in drinks called congeners – the darker the drink the more there are; the direct effect of alcohol and what the liver breaks it down into; dehydration; and low blood sugar are responsible for the well-known symptoms of headache, dizziness, sandpaper mouth, jitters, unsteadiness, nausea, vomiting and indigestion.

Conventional treatment

Sensible drinking in the first place makes a hangover less likely. Drinking water, eating carbohydrates, and vitamin C before retiring to bed may help avoid a hangover. Treatment of a hangover relies on painkillers, indigestion remedies, non-alcoholic liquid to combat dehydration, and food to combat low blood sugar. Milk thistle and artichoke extract help the liver to function well.

Old-fashioned remedies

- **Bananas** – Eat a banana for carbohydrates that help restore depleted sugar levels
- **Cloves** – Chew on one or two cloves and then spit these out
- **Ginger** – Eat fresh, crystallised, in biscuits, or drink ginger tea to relieve nausea
- **Peppermint** – Add a few drops of peppermint oil to olive oil and massage gently into the temples to relieve headache. Alternatively bruise fresh peppermint leaves and apply to the temples. Chew fresh peppermint leaves or drink peppermint tea to freshen the breath
- **Tomato** – Drink a glass of tomato juice for vitamin C to help the liver process alcohol

HAYFEVER

Millions of people suffer sneezing, itchy eyes, and a runny and blocked up nose because of tree or grass pollen allergy, when the body's immune system reacts to pollen mistakenly thinking this is a threat. Some even get itchy ears, an itchy throat, and headaches. Hayfever can also cause wheezing and can leave a person fatigued and miserable because they can't enjoy the summer months.

Conventional treatment

Avoid pollen as best as possible. Hayfever symptoms can be prevented and relieved with antihistamine medication, eye drops and nasal sprays. Some with severe hayfever may be offered immunotherapy to re-educate the immune system.

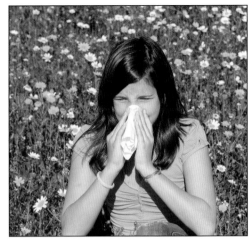

"Hayfever can spoil the summer"

Old-fashioned remedies

- **Apple** – Eat a couple of apples as these contain quercetin, a natural anti-histamine
- **Camomile** – Brew a cup of camomile herb tea, remove the tea bag and allow this to cool until it's at a temperature that can be tolerated and rest it against closed eyes
- **Honey** – A spoonful of honey added to warm water, gargled and swallowed will relieve an itchy throat
- **Steam** – Inhale steam to relieve nasal congestion, and sit in a steamy room to also relieve an itchy throat and soothe itchy eyes
- **Vinegar** – Mix a teaspoon of vinegar with half a cup of water and with the head tilted to one side use a medicine dropper to put a few drops into the ear to relieve itching

HEADACHES

There are many different causes of headaches including stress, dehydration, and hangover. Even taking too many painkillers can result in headaches. The commonest type of headache, however, is a stress, tension, or muscular headache that can be caused by neck and scalp muscle contraction triggered by poor posture, eye strain, and emotional stress. On both sides of the head there's pressure – it sometimes feels like a tight band around the head or a weight pressing down on the top of the head – and pain that's constant and nagging.

Conventional treatment

Painkillers usually relieve headaches, as does relaxation with deep breathing exercises or listening to favourite pieces of music, for example. It's important to get to the bottom of why a headache is happening in the first place and to address this or avoid it as necessary.

"Tension headaches can feel like a tight band around the head"

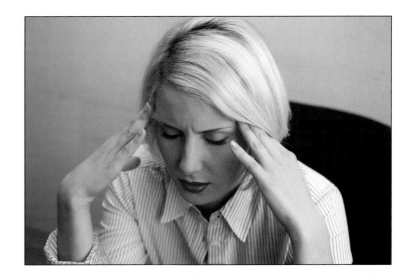

Old-fashioned remedies

- **Bananas** – Make a poultice of ripe banana peel and place against the sore area of the head
- **Camomile** – Drink a cup of camomile tea a few times a day to relieve stress and tension
- **Feverfew** – Make an infusion of the dried leaves and drink this, or eat the leaves in a sandwich
- **Frozen vegetables** – Wrap a bag of frozen vegetables in a soft cloth and place against the scalp where the headache is. It may be easier to lie down and rest the head on the frozen vegetables in the cloth
- **Ginger** – Eat fresh, crystallised, in biscuits, or drink ginger tea
- **Horseradish** – To one tablespoon of finely grated horseradish add half to one tablespoon of water. Wrap in a muslin cloth and apply to the area of the headache. Sniffing freshly grated horseradish can also help
- **Ice** – Wrap some ice in a cloth and apply to the area affected by the headache
- **Lavender** – Add lavender essential oil to a pillow, clothing, or a handkerchief. Inhaling the steam from a hot lavender infusion, drinking this, or adding lavender to a warm bath and soaking in this can all help ease stress
- **Onions** – Place a slice of raw onion on the back of the neck
- **Potato** – Make a potato poultice by boiling one or two large unpeeled potatoes until soft then mash. Remove excess moisture, wrap in a cloth, and place on the back of the neck

Heart disease

Most often the result of narrowed or furred up arteries caused by smoking, high cholesterol, and high blood pressure. This restricts blood flow and contributes to blood clots preventing blood from reaching the heart causing angina or a heart attack. Other diseases affecting the heart include heart failure where the heart becomes too weak to pump blood around the body efficiently and irregular heart beats.

Conventional treatment

Don't smoke and lose weight if needed. Exercise, a low fat diet, and minimal alcohol consumption helps to keep weight, blood pressure and cholesterol at healthy levels. Keep stress under control and eat oily fish each week. Asprin and other medication may be recommended.

Old-fashioned remedies

- **Bananas** – Eat one or two a day as they can help lower blood pressure
- **Garlic** – Consume three to four cloves a day. The allicin in garlic may help lower cholesterol and blood pressure
- **Oats** – Eat plenty as these help lower cholesterol
- **Omega-3** – Consume one to two portions of oily fish a week. Omega-3 essential fatty acids in these decrease the risk of blood clotting, and irregular heart beats, and may lower blood pressure

Hiccups

There's a sudden contraction of the diaphragm and other breathing muscles that quickly draws air into the body. Whilst this is happening an immediate closure of the throat interrupts the intake of air. It's this closure that causes the sound of a hiccup.

Anything that irritates the diaphragm can trigger hiccups, such as stomach distension after eating and drinking too much or too quickly or sudden changes in temperature, for example coming from a warm environment out into the cold air.

For most people with the occasional attack of hiccups there's no obvious reason why they've occurred. If attacks persist longer than usual, or are recurrent, sometimes liver or kidney chemistry imbalance, or an intestinal problem, may be responsible.

Conventional treatment

Everyone has a treatment for hiccups, often passed down from generation to generation. Popular ones include drinking cold water quickly from a glass in the normal way or from the back of the glass, holding the breath and counting to ten, or dropping something cold down a person's back. Relaxation techniques or hypnotherapy can help those suffering with recurrent hiccups too.

Old-fashioned remedies

- **Brown sugar** – Eat a spoonful of brown sugar
- **Ice** – Eat an ice cube or rub this on the outside of the neck over the throat
- **Water** – Drink ice cold water quickly from the back of a glass

HIGH CHOLESTEROL

Cholesterol is essential to the body's metabolism, assisting in the digestive process, and being required for cell membrane manufacture and production of certain hormones. Between twenty-five to thirty-three per cent of the cholesterol found within the body comes from the diet, the remainder being manufactured by the liver.

However, too much cholesterol, specifically low-density lipoprotein (LDL) cholesterol or 'bad' cholesterol, contributes to fatty plaques that fur up the arteries causing heart attacks and stroke, whereas high-density lipoprotein (HDL) cholesterol, or 'good' cholesterol, protects the heart and circulation.

Conventional treatment

Lifestyle changes are an essential component of reducing cholesterol levels. Reducing saturated fat intake, regular exercise, and losing weight where necessary helps lower cholesterol, particularly 'bad' cholesterol, and boosts 'good' cholesterol levels. Medication is also used to reduce high levels of cholesterol.

Old-fashioned remedies

- **Bananas** – Eat one or two a day as they can help lower blood pressure
- **Garlic** – Consume three to four cloves a day. The allicin in garlic may help lower cholesterol and blood pressure
- **Oats** – Eat plenty as these help lower cholesterol
- **Omega-3** – Consume one to two portions of oily fish a week. Omega-3 essential fatty acids in these decrease the risk of blood clotting, irregular heart beats, and may lower blood pressure

IMPETIGO

Impetigo is a highly contagious infection that affects the skin and is mostly caused by the bacterium called staphylococcus aureus. It's easily spread through close contact with someone who already has impetigo.

The infection usually appears around the mouth and nostrils. Initially tiny blisters appear filled with fluid and very soon after these blisters develop into the golden brown crusts that are typical of this infection. Generally those affected remain well but the crusts may feel uncomfortable to the child and look uncomfortable to those around.

Conventional treatment

Fortunately impetigo is easily treated with antibiotics. Since the bacterium can also be spread by sharing towels and cuddling soft toys these need a good boil wash to destroy any bacteria so that reinfection can be prevented.

Old-fashioned remedies

- **Calendula** – Apply as a cream or compress
- **Honey** – Apply honey to the infected areas of skin

INDIGESTION

When stomach acid breaks down the protective stomach lining it causes irritation and inflammation that's felt as indigestion. When acid escapes from the stomach back up into the gullet, called reflux, it causes heartburn and if it reaches the mouth it causes acid regurgitation.

Medicines such as anti-inflammatory drugs can cause indigestion as can eating hot and spicy food and drinking alcohol. Sometimes an infection can cause indigestion, a common one being *Helicobacter pylori* that's responsible for most stomach ulcers that themselves result in painful indigestion.

Being overweight, overeating, wearing tight clothing and being pregnant make acid reflux more likely.

Conventional treatment

Losing weight if needed, not smoking, avoiding food and drink that trigger indigestion, and not eating close to bedtime helps. Antacids that neutralise acid and acid suppressants that reduce production of acid usually quickly relieve symptoms. Antibiotics are used to treat *Helicobacter pylori* infection.

Old-fashioned remedies

- **Bananas** – Eat one banana for its natural antacid benefits
- **Bicarbonate of soda** – Dissolve a level teaspoon in water and drink
- **Lavender** – Drink a cup of lavender tea
- **Lemon balm** – Drink lemon balm tea to relieve stress that can cause indigestion

- **Liquorice** – Take powdered liquorice in water or boil liquorice in hot water and drink the tea
- **Papaya** – Eat the ripe fruit or make into juice and drink
- **Peppermint** – Drink a cup of peppermint tea

INSECT BITES AND STINGS

Common culprits are wasps, bees, ants, mosquitoes or midges. A bite or sting may cause no symptoms at all or may bring up a small red lump, which may or not be itchy or painful.

These are best avoided by being aware of what insects may be around, wearing protective footwear, and using appropriate insect repellent.

Conventional treatment

If the sting is visible it can be removed with tweezers, but avoid squeezing the poison sac as this forces any remaining poison into the skin. Applying a cold compress helps reduce pain and swelling. Sting relief cream and / or calamine cream are often recommended, and painkillers if the affected area is painful.

Old-fashioned remedies

- **Aloe vera** – Apply fresh gel and gently rub in
- **Apple** – Cut an apple in half and then rub it against the bite
- **Bananas** – Rub the inside of a banana peel against the insect bite or sting

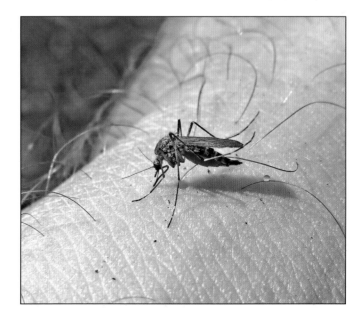

"Bites and stings can be a real irritation"

- **Basil** – Dilute tincture in water in a ratio of 1:5 and apply with a compress
- **Bicarbonate of soda** – Make a paste of bicarbonate of soda and water, spread over the stung area, and leave for five to ten minutes
- **Calendula** – Apply as a tincture, poultice, compress, cream or ointment
- **Horseradish** – Apply a slice of horseradish root to the bite or sting for around twenty to thirty minutes followed by ice for a further five to ten minutes
- **Ice** – Rub an ice cube against the bite or sting for up to a minute, or wrap ice cubes in a cloth and apply to the affected area
- **Lavender** – Make a lavender infusion using the flowers, strain and leave until the temperature is at a level tolerable to the skin. Apply directly to the affected area or as a compress
- **Lemon juice** – Cut a lemon in half and rub the flesh of the lemon against the irritated part
- **Oatmeal** – Make an oatmeal paste by mixing uncooked oatmeal and water, and apply to the itchy area either directly or by placing in muslin cloth
- **Radish** – Cut a slice of radish and rub the white flesh against the bite or sting. Radish juice can also be used for this complaint
- **Tea** – Steep four tea bags in boiling water for ten minutes, allow to cool, then apply liquid to bite or sting using a cloth
- **Vinegar** – Make a mixture of two tablespoons of vinegar with a cup of water and apply to the affected area

INSOMNIA

Most people experience difficulty sleeping at some time in their lives, for a short time or much longer. Physical problems such as pain, emotional problems such as worry, anxiety and depression, and environmental intrusions like noise and an uncomfortable bed are common culprits.

A lack of refreshing sleep also causes tiredness the following day, itself making poor mood and accidents more likely.

Conventional treatment

Sleeping pills are rarely advised to treat insomnia these days except for exceptional circumstances such as bereavement and jet lag. Treatment aims to identify and treat the underlying cause of insomnia, and to get people to practice good sleep hygiene that includes going to bed at a set time, avoiding stimulants before bedtime, and making sure the bedroom is quiet and dark, and the bed comfortable.

Old-fashioned remedies

- **Camomile** – Drink a cup of camomile tea around thirty minutes before bedtime

- **Bay leaf** – Place bay leaves, camomile, and bergamot into a cloth bag and rest head on this to help reduce stress and induce good sleep
- **Lavender** – Add lavender essential oil to a pillow or pyjamas. Inhaling the steam from a hot lavender infusion, drinking this, or adding lavender to a warm bath and soaking in this can all help ease stress
- **Milk** – Drink a cup of warm milk thirty minutes before bedtime

IRRITABLE BOWEL SYNDROME

Irritable bowel syndrome (IBS) is a very common disorder of the gut that can cause abdominal cramping, bloating, diarrhoea and constipation. Its precise cause isn't known but overactivity and oversensitivity of the gut are believed to play a part.

Conventional treatment

Many people benefit from eating more fibre, however, some find this makes things worse. Managing stress helps, as does exercise, cutting down alcohol consumption and not smoking. Medication is used to relieve painful gut spasms, diarrhoea, and constipation. A daily probiotic can be beneficial. Acupuncture, osteopathy, and hypnotherapy can all help to relieve the symptoms of stress and of IBS.

Old-fashioned remedies

- **Aloe vera** – Taking aloe vera juice can ease symptoms of IBS, in particular constipation
- **Camomile** – Drink camomile tea to relieve stress and painful gut spasms
- **Liquorice** – Chew and swallow liquorice or mix half a teaspoon of liquorice root powder with warm water and drink to relieve constipation, gut spasm, bloating, and wind
- **Oatmeal** – A bowl each day helps to avoid constipation
- **Peppermint** – Drink peppermint tea to relieve painful gut spasm and bloating

JOINT PROBLEMS

Joints may swell up, ache, and feel very painful for a number of reasons. Often it's because of an injury such as a twisted or sprained ankle where a ligament is damaged, other times with so many different types of arthritis – osteoarthritis, rheumatoid arthritis, and gout, for example – it's common for one of these to be responsible. The knock on effect means sometimes it's difficult to get on with the day's activities, that's providing it's possible to move about at all.

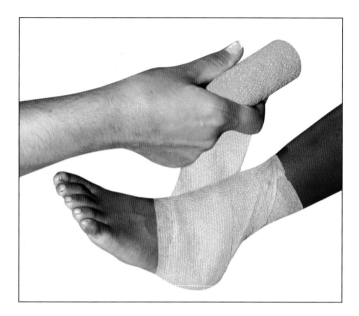

"Sprains can trip up your plans"

Conventional treatment

The RICE technique is recommended for acutely swollen and painful joints – that's Rest, Ice, Compression, and Elevation. This allows the inflammation responsible for the swelling and pain to calm down. Painkillers and anti-inflammatory drugs effectively relieve pain. For long-term joint problems such as arthritis exercise helps relieve pain and strengthen the muscles that support the joint.

Old-fashioned remedies

- **Arnica** – Apply a tincture of arnica to the affected joint or joints with a compress or poultice and fix to the joint with a bandage and leave for fifteen to twenty minutes
- **Basil** – Drink an infusion of basil twice a day
- **Bay leaf** – Tie leaves up in a small muslin cloth and soak in hot water, allow to cool, and then gently rub against the sore area. Alternatively, heat a handful of bay leaves in olive oil for fifteen to twenty minutes, allow to simmer for a further ten minutes, strain the oil, and rub against the affected area once cool enough to do so
- **Feverfew** – Soak a clean cloth in a freshly brewed feverfew infusion and apply to the affected joint. If more than one joint is affected it may be simpler to consume a cup of weak feverfew tea
- **Figs** – Soak four figs in water and then mash these into a poultice. Apply directly to the affected area and keep in place with a clean cloth or dressing. Leave for thirty minutes to an hour
- **Frozen vegetables** – Place a bag of these wrapped in a cloth against the affected area

- **Ginger** – Drink ginger tea once or twice a day
- **Horseradish** – Boil a cup of milk and mix in two tablespoons of grated horseradish. Soak a clean cloth in the mixture and apply to the affected area. The mixture when cooled to a tolerable temperature can also be massaged into the sore joint
- **Ice** – Apply ice wrapped in cloth to the affected area
- **Lavender** – Make a compress and apply to the affected areas
- **Lemon balm** – Soak a clean dressing in an infusion of lemon balm and apply to the affected joint as a warm, or cold, compress
- **Potato** – Boil chopped up new potatoes, strain, and soak a cloth in broth and apply to affected joint
- **Thyme** – Make thyme tea, allow to cool, soak a clean cloth in it, and apply to affected area for ten to fifteen minutes
- **Turmeric** – Make a paste and apply to the affected area, fixing in place with cling film, or a dressing
- **Vinegar** – Rub warmed vinegar into the affected joint

LARYNGITIS

This simply means inflammation of the larynx, or voice box. It's most often caused by a viral infection at the same time as a cough and cold, commonly resulting in a painful throat, a croaky or hoarse voice, difficulty speaking, or even losing the voice for up to a week. Allergy can also cause laryngitis. For those who smoke or sing laryngitis can last much longer, sometimes months.

Conventional treatment

There's no specific treatment as the body will sort things out itself. Whilst this is happening it's important to rest the voice, and relieve symptoms with painkillers and anti-inflammatory medication, gargling to soothe any accompanying sore throat and drinking plenty of liquid.

Old-fashioned remedies

- **Basil** – Make a decoction of basil leaves by mashing the leaves and then boiling these in water. Ginger and honey can be added if desired. Allow to cool and then drink

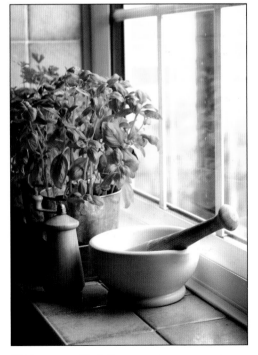

"A king amongst herbs"

- **Bay leaf** – Make a poultice of bay leaves after boiling these in water. When cool enough apply directly to the outside of the throat and leave for up to thirty minutes
- **Garlic** – Chew a clove of garlic each day until the sore throat has resolved
- **Ginger** – Finely grate fresh ginger into a cup and add boiling water, allow to cool to a comfortable temperature, then gargle and swallow. Honey and lemon juice can be added
- **Honey** – Eat a spoonful of honey. Alternatively to warm water add a spoonful of honey and a squeeze of lemon juice, mix these together, then gargle and swallow
- **Lemon juice** – Mix one tablespoon of lemon juice in a cup of hot water, allow to cool to a comfortable temperature, then gargle and swallow. Honey can be added
- **Liquorice** – Mix powdered liquorice root with warm water, then gargle, and swallow
- **Peppermint** – Breath in the steam of hot water with peppermint oil added through the mouth taking care not to get too close to avoid the mouth getting burned
- **Vinegar** – Mix one tablespoon of vinegar in warm water, gargle then swallow. Honey and lemon can be added

LEG CRAMPS

Many people experience leg cramps, painful spasms of the muscles, and most often these occur during or after exercise or strenuous activity. Cramps can also occur when a muscle is injured, when sweating a lot due to loss of salt and water, and when furred up arteries prevent sufficient oxygen getting through to the muscles. Nocturnal leg cramps wake people up and prevent good sleep.

Conventional treatment

As with many health complaints getting to the root cause of the problem and treating this eliminates the leg cramps. Stretching before exercise helps prevent cramps, as does drinking enough water particularly when sweating a lot. Quinine sulphate tablets are recommended to prevent nocturnal leg cramps. Not smoking and keeping blood pressure and cholesterol at safe levels lessens the risk of narrowed arteries.

Old-fashioned remedies

- **Feverfew** – Make an infusion of the dried leaves and drink this or eat the leaves in a sandwich to relieve cramps caused by inflammation
- **Ginger** – Drink ginger tea once or twice a day to relieve cramps caused by inflammation
- **Tonic water** – Drink up to a glass of tonic water before bedtime to prevent nocturnal leg cramps

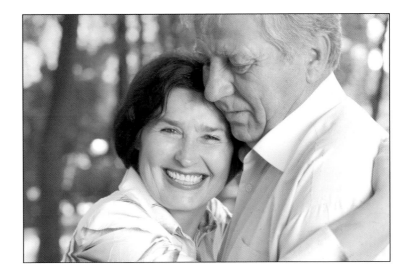

"Making time for each other helps bring back libido"

Poor libido

Poor libido or decreased sex drive is a loss of interest in sex. The fast-paced, high-pressured lives that many people lead causing tiredness and stress are usually responsible. Other causes include anaemia, under-active thyroid gland, depression, medication side effects, relationship problems, in women the menopause and in men low testosterone and erection difficulties.

Conventional treatment

The aim is to identify the underlying cause and sort this out. Exercise, relaxation, not becoming overtired, cutting down alcohol consumption whilst increasing consumption of energy-boosting B vitamins and libido boosting zinc and ginseng, can all help libido. Talking about the problem either with your partner, doctor, or a sex therapist helps.

Old-fashioned remedies

- **Camomile** – Drink a cup of camomile tea a few times a day to relieve stress and tension
- **Lavender** – Add lavender essential oil to a pillow, clothing, or a handkerchief. Inhaling the steam from a hot lavender infusion, drinking this, or adding lavender to a warm bath and soaking in this can all help ease stress
- **Onions** – Eat half an onion a day

Migraine

It's thought that an imbalance in activity of brain chemicals is responsible for migraine, a specific type of headache, where blood vessels become dilated and inflamed resulting in severe throbbing and incapacitating pain that's usually felt on one side of the head and is often accompanied by nausea, vomiting and a dislike of bright lights, noise, and smells. For some people the headache is preceded by an aura of visual disturbances, numbness and pins and needles, speech problems, or other odd sensations like sensing odd smells, for example.

Migraine is often triggered by stress, missed or delayed meals, tiredness, dehydration, menstrual periods, glaring or flickering lights, and certain foods and drinks such as cheese, chocolate, alcohol, tea, and coffee.

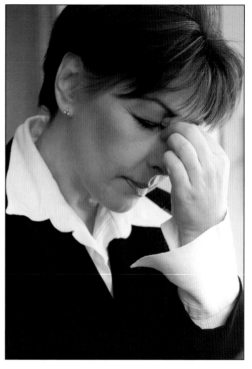

Conventional treatment

Avoid identified triggers, eat regularly, avoid tiredness, and get plenty of rest and relaxation. Migraine attacks are treated with painkillers, anti-inflammatory drugs, anti-sickness drugs, or specific migraine medication. Medication can also be used to prevent recurrent migraine attacks.

"Migraine imprisons someone in a quiet dark room"

Old-fashioned remedies

- **Bananas** – Make a poultice of ripe banana peel and place against the sore area of the head
- **Feverfew** – Make an infusion of the dried leaves and drink this, or eat the leaves in a sandwich
- **Frozen vegetables** – Wrap a bag of frozen vegetables in a cloth and place against the scalp where the headache is. It may be easier to lie down and rest the head on the frozen vegetables in the cloth
- **Ginger** – Eat fresh, crystallised, in biscuits, or drink ginger tea
- **Horseradish** – To one tablespoon of finely grated horseradish add half to one tablespoon of water. Wrap in a muslin cloth and apply to the area of the headache. Sniffing freshly grated horseradish can also help
- **Ice** – Wrap some ice in a clean cloth and apply to the area affected by the headache
- **Lavender** – Make a lavender infusion and inhale the steam. Drinking the lavender tea can also help
- **Onions** – Place a slice of raw onion on the back of the neck

- **Potato** – Make a potato poultice by boiling one or two large unpeeled potatoes until soft then mash. Remove excess moisture, wrap in a cloth, and place on the back of the neck

MORNING SICKNESS

This occurs in pregnancy, often being a thing of the past by around fourteen weeks. That said some women suffer nausea and vomiting throughout their pregnancy, and not always in the morning. Why it happens is not known but pregnancy hormones are thought to play a part.

Conventional treatment

Reassurance that morning sickness will not harm an unborn baby, and for most women will be over by around fourteen weeks of pregnancy, together with simple advice to eat bite-size portions of dry and bland foods, eating little and often, and avoiding foods and smells that triggers attacks of nausea is usually all that's needed. Ginger is commonly recommended as is wearing wrist acupressure bands. Sometimes medication may be advised. When vomiting is severe admission to hospital for intravenous rehydration may be needed.

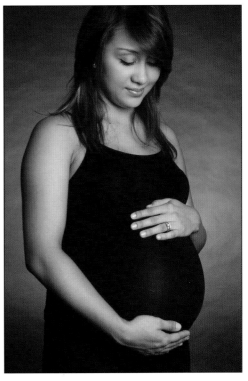

"Morning sickness can wipe away the bloom of pregnancy"

Old-fashioned remedies

- **Bananas** – Eat sliced banana slowly, eating according to symptoms
- **Ginger** – Eat fresh, crystallised, in biscuits or drink ginger tea
- **Lavender** – Drink a cup of lavender tea
- **Onions** – Place a slice of raw onion under each armpit
- **Peppermint** – Drink peppermint tea

MOUTH ULCERS

Accidental gum damage by teeth or tooth brushing, for example, or being rundown and stressed are the commonest causes of mouth ulcers, which are often painful. Other less common causes include immune disorders, and vitamin and mineral deficiencies.

Conventional treatment

The usual approach is to use pastilles or gels containing anaesthetic to relieve pain whilst the ulcer is healing. Rinsing the mouth with ice-cold water before eating numbs the pain and makes eating more comfortable. Vitamin C, the B vitamins, iron, and zinc will keep the immune system strong since recurrent mouth ulcers often occur when the body is run down. When necessary, nutritional deficiencies are corrected with an appropriate diet or supplementation. Practising good dental hygiene and keeping stress to a minimum should help to keep mouth ulcers at bay.

Old-fashioned remedies

- **Basil** – Make a decoction or infusion of basil leaves with boiling water. Allow to cool and then rinse around mouth before either spitting out or swallowing the liquid
- **Camomile** – Allow a cup of camomile herb tea to cool and then use as a mouth rinse. In can help to make up a container or jug of camomile tea, and store in the fridge ready to use when needed
- **Ginger** – Cut a slice of ginger, crush between fingers and press against the mouth ulcer
- **Honey** – After washing the hands rub some honey gently against the ulcer. Alternatively, take a spoonful of honey into the mouth and rub it against the ulcer with the tongue
- **Ice** – Suck and roll an ice cube around the mouth ulcer
- **Liquorice** – Suck and roll liquorice around the mouth ulcer
- **Salt** – Place salt directly against the ulcer. Alternatively make a solution of a cup of warm water with a third of a level teaspoon of salt and rinse around the mouth, spitting it out afterwards
- **Tea** – Add four to six tea bags to boiling water, leave to steep for ten minutes, then allow to cool to a comfortable temperature to enable the liquid to be used as mouthwash but not swallowed

MUSCLE PROBLEMS

Muscles may swell up, ache, and feel very painful for a number of reasons. Often it's because of a sudden injury such as a groin strain, sometimes it's because of repetitive strain injury where a muscle has been used over and over again and gradually a problem has developed. These muscle problems often occur because they have not been warmed up sufficiently before being used. Sometimes side effects of medication may also be responsible. Consequently it can be difficult to get on with the day's activities.

Conventional treatment

The RICE technique can be used to treat acutely swollen and painful muscles – that's Rest, Ice, Compression, and Elevation. This allows the inflammation responsible for the swelling and pain to calm down. Painkillers and anti-inflammatory drugs effectively relieve pain as can massage.

Old-fashioned remedies

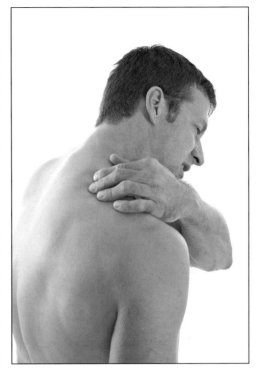

"Stress, injury or an uncomfortable bed can be a pain in the neck"

- **Arnica** – Apply a tincture of arnica to the affected muscle or muscles with a compress or poultice and fix to the muscle with a bandage and leave for fifteen to twenty minutes
- **Basil** – Drink an infusion of basil twice a day
- **Bay leaf** – Tie leaves up in a small muslin cloth and soak in hot water, allow to cool, and then gently rub against the sore area. Alternatively, heat a handful of bay leaves in olive oil for fifteen to twenty minutes, allow to simmer for a further ten minutes, strain the oil, and rub against the affected area once cool enough to do so
- **Epsom salts** – Add a few tablespoons of Epsom salts to warm bath water and relax. Alternatively, make a paste of Epsom salts with hot water and apply to the affected area. Leave for ten to fifteen minutes and then wash off well
- **Feverfew** – Soak a clean cloth in a freshly brewed feverfew infusion and apply to the affected muscle. If more than one muscle is affected it may be simpler to consume a cup of weak feverfew tea
- **Figs** – Soak four figs in water and then mash these into a poultice. Apply directly to the affected area and keep in place with a clean cloth or dressing. Leave for thirty minutes to an hour
- **Frozen vegetables** – Place a bag of these wrapped in a cloth against the affected area
- **Ginger** – Drink ginger tea once or twice a day
- **Horseradish** – Boil a cup of milk and mix in two tablespoons of grated horseradish. Soak a clean cloth in the mixture and apply to the affected area. The mixture when cooled to a tolerable temperature can also be massaged into the sore muscle
- **Ice** – Apply ice wrapped in cloth to the affected area
- **Lavender** – Make a compress and apply to the affected areas

- **Lemon balm** – Soak a clean dressing in an infusion of lemon balm and apply to the affected muscle as a warm, or cold, compress
- **Peppermint** – Allow a cup of peppermint tea to cool and then soak a clean cloth with this. Press against the affected muscle and hold in place with a bandage
- **Potato** – Boil chopped up new potatoes, strain, and soak cloth in broth and apply to affected area
- **Thyme** – Make thyme tea, allow to cool, soak a clean cloth in it, and apply to affected area for ten to fifteen minutes
- **Turmeric** – Make a paste and apply to the affected area, fixing in place with cling film, or a dressing
- **Vinegar** – Rub warmed vinegar into the affected muscle
- **Witch hazel** – Apply as tea, tincture, or a cream to the affected muscle

NASAL CONGESTION

A blocked and stuffy nose is common with cough and cold infections. It can also be caused by sinusitis or allergy, such as hayfever or perennial allergic rhinitis. Inflammation causes swelling and excess mucus to be produced that in turn narrow the nasal passages and block the channels connecting the sinuses to the nasal passages preventing drainage of mucus.

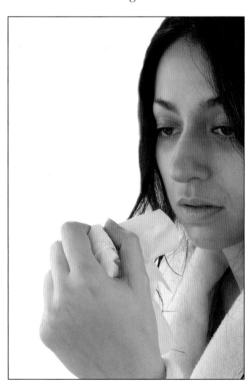

"You may sound funny to others but being bunged up is no fun"

Nasal congestion makes breathing difficult, changes the quality of the voice, and increases the likelihood of snoring.

Conventional treatment

Steam inhalation, painkillers, decongestant nasal sprays or drops, and saline or seawater nasal sprays can help to relieve symptoms. Some benefit from using an ioniser or a humidifier to moisten the air in the room. Sometimes surgery is required to drain the sinuses or remove any tissue that is contributing to congestion.

Old-fashioned remedies

- **Aloe vera** – Boil one or two leaves in water and then inhale the steam
- **Garlic** – Chew fresh garlic increasing the amount as needed
- **Ginger** – Inhale steam from hot ginger tea before drinking

- **Horseradish** – Slice horseradish root and breathe in deeply or chew slices of horseradish beginning with a small slice increasing the amount as needed
- **Lemon balm** – Drink lemon balm tea after inhaling the steam
- **Onions** – Chew a small slice of fresh onion increasing the amount as needed
- **Peppermint** – Inhale the steam from hot water with peppermint oil added taking care not to scald the nostrils
- **Radish** – Chew a red globe radish
- **Salt** – Make a mixture of two cups of warm water and half a teaspoon of salt. Apply this to the nasal passages on a cotton bud soaked in the mixture, or by using a dropper to squirt mixture into the nose. Alternatively sniff the solution from a small glass into the nostril whilst keeping the other nostril closed

NAUSEA AND VOMITING

There's no getting away from the fact that nausea and vomiting are not pleasant. This is commonly accompanied by diarrhoea when caused by infection that 'does the rounds' and food poisoning. Pregnancy morning sickness, travel, hangover, side effects of drugs and treatments such as chemotherapy, anxiety and stress may also cause nausea and vomiting.

Conventional treatment

Usually time is the healer as the body clears any infection or the trigger, travel for example, is over. Until this time anti-sickness medication, acupressure, and light foods can help. Sipping water is important to maintain hydration whilst minimising the chance of triggering vomiting.

Old-fashioned remedies

- **Basil** – Make an infusion of basil in boiling water, allow to cool, and then drink
- **Cloves** – Chew on one or two cloves and then spit these out
- **Ginger** – Eat fresh, crystallised, in biscuits or drink ginger tea
- **Lavender** – Drink a cup of lavender tea
- **Onions** – Place a slice of raw onion under each armpit
- **Peppermint** – Drink peppermint tea

NEURALGIA

This is the severe pain that originates from a nerve. One type, called trigeminal neuralgia, causes severe pain usually on one side of the face, and results from pressure on a nerve. Another common type occurs after shingles infection, called post-herpetic neuralgia, and is felt where the shingles rash appeared.

Neuralgia pain spasms may occur throughout the day, everyday, but may disappear for months or years before recurring. Severe pain like this brings people down very quickly making them depressed and sometimes unable to perform everyday activities.

Conventional treatment

The aim is to bring the pain under control. Standard painkillers are often not effective and more potent ones, and drugs that are usually used to treat other conditions such as epilepsy and depression but which can relieve pain too, are needed. Sometimes surgery, injections and other treatments are used to block or numb the nerves. With neuralgia it's important to get emotional support too.

Old-fashioned remedies

- **Arnica** – Apply a cold compress or a warm poultice to the affected area
- **Calendula** – Apply as a tincture, poultice, compress, cream or ointment
- **Feverfew** – Make an infusion of dried leaves, and allow this to cool. Then apply to the affected area as a compress
- **Potato** – Bake a potato, immediately wrap in a cloth to maintain its warmth, and gently place against sore area of skin. Potato can be mashed soft if desired
- **Witch hazel** – Soak a cotton wool ball or clean cloth in witch hazel tea and apply to the affected area

NOSEBLEEDS

Usually the result of a minor injury, or overenthusiastic nose blowing or picking, they can also occur when nasal infection causes the lining of the nostrils to become dry and cracked.

Conventional treatment

Sit down and firmly pinch the soft part of the nose, just above the nostrils, together for ten minutes. Lean forward breathing through the mouth. Allow blood to clot by maintaining the pressure on the nose for fifteen minutes. If bleeding cannot be stopped then seek medical advice.

Old-fashioned remedies

- **Frozen vegetables** – Wrap a bag of frozen vegetables in a soft cloth, and apply to the bridge of the nose
- **Ice** – Wrap ice cubes in a soft cloth, and apply to the bridge of the nose
- **Lemon juice** – Soak cotton wool in lemon juice and put into nostril

PALPITATIONS

These are irregular or rapid heartbeats often described as pounding, thumping, or racing. Stress or stimulants such as caffeine and alcohol may be responsible, as may medication side effects. Sometimes palpitations are caused by a heart condition, or other medical conditions such as anaemia, an overactive thyroid gland, panic attacks, or depression.

Conventional treatment

Avoid any palpitation triggers, such as caffeine and keep stress under control. Treatment aims to eliminate any underlying cause such as a heart condition or anaemia.

Old-fashioned remedies

- **Camomile** – Drink a cup of camomile tea a few times a day to relieve stress and tension
- **Lavender** – Add lavender essential oil to a pillow, clothing, or a handkerchief. Inhaling the steam from a hot lavender infusion, drinking this, or adding lavender to a warm bath and soaking in this can all help ease stress
- **Lemon balm** – Drink warm lemon balm tea a couple of times a day to relieve anxiety

PERIOD PAIN

Period pains may be caused by infection, fibroids or endometriosis. However, most often there's no disease of the womb and the cause of painful periods, also known as menstrual cramps, remains unclear, but possibly related to a build up of normal body chemicals called prostaglandins or an oversensitivity of the womb to these.

Conventional treatment

A hot water bottle provides warmth and pain relief as does a hot bath. Painkillers and anti-inflammatory medication also relieve pain and the oral contraceptive pill makes period pain and heavy periods less likely. If period pain has an identified cause, for example endometriosis, this can be treated.

Old-fashioned remedies

- **Brown sugar** – Add brown sugar to ginger tea and consume a couple of times a day
- **Cabbage** – Place chilled cabbage leaves against the lower abdomen and leave for a couple of hours. Alternatively, warm up the leaves first by blanching in boiling water, running a hot iron over them, or putting them in a microwave
- **Camomile** – Drink a cup of camomile tea a few times a day to relieve stress and tension
- **Feverfew** – Drink a weak infusion of feverfew

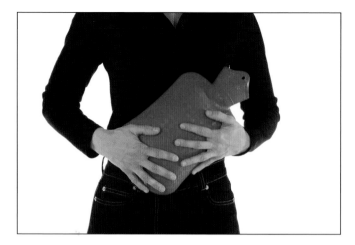

"A hot water bottle is comforting"

- **Ginger** – Eat grated fresh ginger, crystallised, or drink ginger tea
- **Lavender** – Add lavender essential oil to a pillow, clothing, or a handkerchief. Inhaling the steam from a hot lavender infusion, drinking this, or adding lavender to a warm bath and soaking in this can all help ease stress

PREMENSTRUAL SYNDROME (PMS)

Symptoms of PMS usually happen at the same time each month, anytime up to two weeks before a period starts. Common ones are feeling irritable, bad-tempered, upset or emotional; mood swings; fluid retention and feeling bloated; breast tenderness; and changes to the skin and hair. PMS symptoms usually ease off once the period starts and then disappear until the cycle begins again.

PMS is believed to be linked to changing levels of female hormones during the menstrual cycle but the precise cause isn't known.

Conventional treatment

Lifestyle changes help such as exercise and cutting down on salt, caffeine and alcohol. Vitamin B6, vitamin E, magnesium, agnus cactus, and evening primrose oil help overall symptoms of PMS. Medication can be used including non-steroidal anti-inflammatory drugs to ease pain and discomfort, antispasmodic drugs to relieve stomach cramps, the contraceptive pill to stabilise hormone levels, diuretics to relieve bloating and fluid retention, and anti-depressants when PMS is severe.

Old-fashioned remedies

- **Cabbage** – Place chilled cabbage leaves against the affected breast to relieve breast tenderness or the lower abdomen to relieve abdominal pains and leave for a couple of hours. Alternatively, warm up the leaves first by blanching in boiling water, running a hot iron over them, or putting them in a microwave

- **Camomile** – Drink a cup of camomile tea a few times a day to relieve stress and tension
- **Coconut oil** – Take one to two teaspoons of coconut oil on the days when PMS symptoms usually occur
- **Feverfew** – Drink a weak infusion of feverfew on the days leading up to a period
- **Ginger** – Eat grated fresh ginger, crystallised, or drink ginger tea
- **Lavender** – Add lavender essential oil to a pillow, clothing, or a handkerchief. Inhaling the steam from a hot lavender infusion, drinking this, or adding lavender to a warm bath and soaking in this can all help ease stress
- **Liquorice** – Take powdered liquorice root in warm water
- **Onion** – Eat half an onion on the days leading up to a period

PRICKLY HEAT

This irritating itchy red rash, which causes a prickling sensation and is also known as heat rash or miliaria, most often occurs during hot weather when excess sweating makes it easier for bacteria and dead skin cells to block the sweat glands. Sweat gets trapped under the skin where it irritates the skin causing a red, spotty rash, and prickly sensation. Those who sweat a lot or who are overweight, and babies because their sweat glands are not yet fully developed, are most likely to develop prickly heat.

Conventional treatment

Prickly heat clears within a few days. In the meantime keep the skin cool with cool water and by remaining in a cool environment, wear loose cotton clothing that's less likely to irritate the skin, and creams such as hydrocortisone and calamine are used to relieve itching.

Old-fashioned remedies

- **Aloe vera** – Apply fresh gel to the affected area and gently rub in
- **Apple** – Cut an apple in half and then rub it against the skin
- **Bicarbonate of soda** – Mix bicarbonate of soda and water and apply to affected area
- **Carrots** – Apply freshly cut slices of carrot to the itchy areas
- **Cucumber** – Place a slice of cucumber against the sore skin or grind cucumber into a paste and then apply to sore area of skin
- **Horseradish** – Juice slices of horseradish and add to honey then apply to the affected areas
- **Ice** – Apply ice wrapped in cloth to the affected area
- **Milk** – Add a tablespoon of salt to a cup of milk, mix together, then apply to affected area, and leave to dry

- **Oatmeal** – Make an oatmeal paste by mixing uncooked oatmeal and water, and apply to the itchy areas either directly or by placing in muslin cloth
- **Olive oil** – Pour some into the palm of the hand and gently massage into the skin
- **Potato** – Grate a potato and apply as a poultice

PSORIASIS

Psoriasis is a common skin condition that occurs when the skin replaces itself too quickly. Normally skin cells turnover in twenty-one to twenty-eight days, in psoriasis new skin cells appear in just two to six days. This rapid turnover of cells in psoriasis causes itchy red scaly patches, topped with silvery scales, to appear on the skin – most often these patches appear on the elbows, knees, and scalp but they can appear anywhere on the body.

Psoriasis is not contagious and is not caused by poor hygiene. It can cause a form of arthritis and damage the nails.

Psoriasis is thought to be an autoimmune disease, one where for an unexplained reason the immune system turns on the skin cells. It's not clear precisely why this happens. Psoriasis can run in families and often follows infections, periods of stress, or anything that damages the skin.

Conventional treatment

Psoriasis can't be cured but can be kept under control with creams, ointments, and lotions, mousse and gels, phototherapy, and medication.

Old-fashioned remedies

- **Aloe vera** – Apply fresh gel to the affected area and gently rub in
- **Apple** – Cut an apple in half and then rub it against the skin
- **Carrots** – Apply freshly cut slices of carrot to the itchy areas
- **Cucumber** – Place a slice of cucumber against the sore skin or grind cucumber into a paste and then apply to sore area of skin
- **Ice** – Apply ice wrapped in cloth to the affected area
- **Oatmeal** – Make an oatmeal paste by mixing uncooked oatmeal and water, and apply to the itchy areas either directly or by placing in muslin cloth
- **Potato** – Rub the flesh of half a potato against affected area or grate a potato and apply as a poultice
- **Salt** – Mix one cup of warm water with one third of a teaspoon of sea salt. Soak a cotton bud or piece of tissue in the mixture and apply to the affected area
- **Turmeric** – Mix together coconut oil with turmeric powder and gently apply to the affected area

Raynaud's phenomenon

In this common disorder the small blood vessels in the extremities – fingers, toes, ears, tip of nose – are oversensitive to changes in temperature. Exposure to cold, or even a small change in temperature, for example, putting the hands into the fridge, or any stress, interrupts the blood supply to the extremities. The skin turns white, then for some people blue, and then finally red, and at this stage the pain, numbness, and tingling occur.

Conventional treatment

Not smoking and eating a low fat diet helps keep the blood vessels healthy. Exercise stimulates the circulation and keeping warm helps to prevent the blood vessels from constricting. If Raynaud's is mild keeping warm and using hand warmers, for example, and gloves when taking things from the fridge or freezer, may be all that's needed. When it's more severe drugs are available that keep the blood vessels dilated for example. Taking gingko biloba can help.

Old-fashioned remedies

- **Garlic** – Consume three to four cloves a day. The allicin helps to keep the circulation healthy
- **Ginger** – Eat fresh, crystallised, in biscuits, or drink ginger tea, as ginger is a body warmer
- **Omega-3** – Consume one to two portions of oily fish a week. Omega-3 essential fatty acids in these keep the circulation healthy
- **Potato** – Put a hot baked potato wrapped in foil in the coat pocket as a hand warmer. Once cooled eat it

Razor burn

Using a blunt blade to shave any part of the body, or not shaving properly, can result in a rash, called razor burn. Sometimes the rash feels a little uncomfortable and if it's severe small bumps appear too that may become infected pustules. Usually the rash resolves within a matter of hours to days.

Conventional treatment

Avoid it in the first place by using a sharp blade and a good technique to shave – not using too much pressure, plenty of lubrication to keep the skin moist, and shaving in the direction of hair growth. An aftershave cream will soothe any sting and skin soreness. If infection is present then antibiotic treatment may be needed.

Old-fashioned remedies

- **Aloe vera** – Apply fresh aloe vera gel to the affected area and gently rub in
- **Cold water** – Splash this onto face
- **Cucumber** – Place a slice of cucumber against the sore skin or grind cucumber into a paste and then apply to sore area of skin
- **Ice** – Apply ice wrapped in cloth to the affected area
- **Witch hazel** – Apply to the skin with a cotton wool ball or clean cloth soaked in witch hazel tea
- **Yogurt** – Apply directly to the skin, allow to dry and leave for ten to fifteen minutes, before rinsing off with cool water

RINGWORM

Despite its name ringworm is not caused by a worm. It's actually caused by a fungus that infects the skin anywhere on the body including the scalp and the nails. When on the skin the rash is red, scaly, and itchy, and heals from the centre so creating the appearance of a red-ring – hence its name.

The fungi that cause ringworm can be passed on from people and animals with the infection, and from inanimate objects contaminated with the fungal sores.

Conventional treatment

Ringworm on the body is treated with an antifungal cream.

Old-fashioned remedies

- **Garlic** – Crush two cloves of garlic and apply to the affected area
- **Papaya** – Apply papaya sliced, mashed, or as a juice. Massage into the skin and allow it to dry. Leave for ten minutes and then rinse off gently with cool or warm water
- **Turmeric** – Make a paste by mixing two tablespoons of turmeric into boiling water. Add one tablespoon of lemon or lime juice if desired. Apply paste to the affected areas with a clean cloth and leave for twenty to thirty minutes. Hold in place by taping the cloth or by using cling film if possible. Do this twice a day
- **Vinegar** – Soak a cotton wool ball in vinegar and apply to the affected area. The cotton wool can be taped to the affected area and left overnight

SEBORRHOEIC DERMATITIS

This is also known as seborrhoeic eczema and arises when too much sebum, the oily liquid that stops the hair and skin drying out, is produced by the sebaceous glands in the skin. Together with dead skin cells the excess sebum clogs up the pores forming the thick, yellow, greasy scales, or bad dandruff on the scalp, face, the outer ear canal, and the eyelids. It sometimes causes a red rash on these parts of the body too, and may be itchy.

It is not because of poor hygiene and is not infectious. It's common in teenagers and young adults.

Conventional treatment

Treatment is with an antidandruff or anti-fungal shampoo or an anti-fungal cream. Don't pick the scabs as this may damage the skin.

Old-fashioned remedies

- **Olive oil** – Massage olive oil into the scalp and leave overnight. The following morning gently rinse the hair. Do this daily until problem has cleared
- **Turmeric** – Mix turmeric with hot water, add a teaspoon of lemon juice, and massage into affected area. Leave for up to thirty minutes and then wash off
- **Vinegar** – Soak the scalp and hair with vinegar, leave for an hour or so, and then rinse

SKIN IRRITATION

The largest organ of the body the skin can become sore, itchy, and irritated for many reasons. Eczema, psoriasis, allergy, infection, exposure to cold and hot weather, stress, and a less than healthy diet with too little water can all be reflected in the skin, making it red, sore, and dull looking.

Conventional treatment

Keeping the body hydrated and the skin moisturised are the foundations of healthy skin. Skin needs vitamins C and E and needs to be kept out of the way of too much UV radiation and known skin irritants. Medicated creams, lotions, and ointments are used as appropriate.

Old-fashioned remedies

- **Aloe vera** – Apply fresh aloe vera gel to the affected area and gently rub in
- **Apples** – Cut an apple in half and then rub it against the skin
- **Bicarbonate of soda** – Mix bicarbonate of soda and water and apply to affected area
- **Calendula** – Apply as a tincture, poultice, compress, cream or ointment
- **Carrots** – Apply freshly cut slices of carrot to the itchy areas
- **Coconut oil** – Apply to the affected area. Turmeric can be mixed with the coconut oil if desired
- **Cucumber** – Place a slice of cucumber against the sore skin or grind cucumber into a paste and then apply to sore area of skin

- **Frozen vegetables** – Place a bag of these wrapped in a cloth against the affected area
- **Horseradish** – Juice slices of horseradish and add to honey then apply to the affected areas
- **Ice** – Apply ice wrapped in cloth to the affected area
- **Milk** – Add a tablespoon of salt to a cup of milk, mix together, then apply to affected area, and leave to dry
- **Oatmeal** – Make an oatmeal paste by mixing uncooked oatmeal and water, and apply to the itchy areas either directly or by placing in muslin cloth
- **Olive oil** – Pour some into the palm of the hand and gently massage into the skin
- **Potato** – Rub the flesh of half a potato against affected area or grate a potato and apply as a poultice
- **Tea** – Steep four tea bags in boiling water for ten minutes. Allow to cool, and then apply liquid to the affected area using a cloth
- **Tomato** – Puree peeled tomatoes and add to a spoonful of yogurt or a spoonful of buttermilk and then apply. Alternatively slice the tomatoes, dip in yogurt or buttermilk and apply to affected areas
- **Turmeric** – Mix together coconut oil with turmeric powder and gently apply to the affected area
- **Vinegar** – Mix two tablespoons of vinegar with a cup of water and apply to affected area
- **Witch hazel** – Apply to the skin with a cotton wool ball or clean cloth soaked in witch hazel tea
- **Yogurt** – Apply directly to the skin, allow to dry and leave for ten to fifteen minutes, before rinsing off with cool water

SNORING

Snoring occurs when the roof of the mouth and other tissues in the nose and mouth vibrate because air flow through them is not smooth. Snoring disturbs those around the snorer, but also affects the snorer because of obstructive sleep apnoea, when a person repeatedly stops breathing for a few seconds causing them to wake up at night, leaving them tired the following day.

Anything that relaxes the airways, such as alcohol, or that puts pressure on the neck, such as excess fat, makes snoring more likely. Physical obstruction to smooth airflow such as nasal swelling and congestion due to allergy, smoking, a deviated nasal septum, or nasal polyps increases the chance of snoring. Mouth breathers are more likely to snore when sleeping as are those who sleep on their back.

Conventional treatment

Reduce alcohol consumption and lose weight, and treat underlying problems such as allergy. Encouraging sleeping on the side rather than the back, by sewing a tennis ball into a pyjama top for example, means someone is less likely to snore. There are many self-help treatments including nasal strips and jaw repositioning devices. Try Olbas or eucalyptus oil on pillowcase to help keep nasal passages clear. Sometimes surgery is needed.

Old-fashioned remedies

- **Peppermint** – Inhale steam with peppermint oil added taking care not to get too close to avoid the nasal passages getting burned
- **Rolling pin** – Place the rolling pin next to the person whilst they sleep on their side or put it inside the pyjama top, loose or sewn in
- **Steam** – Inhale this before going to bed. Menthol, Olbas, or eucalyptus oil can be added

SORE EYES

Eye strain may cause sore eyes and can indicate that it's time for an eye test to see if glasses, contact lenses, or a new prescription of these is necessary. Sore eyes also occur with hayfever, infection, and if something gets into the eyes that shouldn't be there. Sometimes the eyes feel sore when a person is just overtired or stressed. Eyes can feel sore if they've been exposed to too much UV light too.

Conventional treatment

This depends on what's causing the soreness but usually involves treatment with eye drops to treat infection and allergy, or artificial tears if dryness is causing the eyes to be sore. Resting the eyes is important, as is wearing glasses or contact lenses if needed.

Like the skin, eyes too need protecting from UV light with sunglasses, and relaxing often relieves sore eyes as does bathing them.

Old-fashioned remedies

- **Camomile** – Brew a cup of camomile tea, remove the tea bag and allow to cool until it's at a temperature that can be tolerated and rest it against closed eyes
- **Cucumber** – Place a chilled slice of cucumber over the closed eyelids
- **Papaya** – Make a poultice of mashed papaya fruit and place over closed eyes
- **Potato** – Extract juice from one or two potatoes, soak cotton wool in the juice, and gently hold against closed eyes
- **Tea** – Add a tea bag to boiled water, leave for around five minutes and then remove, squeeze out and allow to cool to a tolerable temperature then place over closed eyes
- **Thyme** – Make a compress of thyme tea and place gently over closed eyes

SORE THROAT

Sore throats are very common. Coughs and colds, tonsillitis, and glandular fever infections are often responsible as is overuse of the throat, for example, when singing.

Some medicines, for example, inhaled steroids, can leave the throat feeling dry and uncomfortable. Anxiety, environmental pollutants, allergy, and acid reflux can also make the throat feel sore, scratchy, itchy, and leave the voice hoarse.

Conventional treatment

Ease the soreness by gargling with salt water, and with warm honey and lemon drinks. Painkiller and anti-inflammatory medication relieves pain and soreness. Treating any underlying condition resolves the problem. For example, when bacteria are responsible then antibiotics will be recommended, if an allergy is responsible then allergy treatments will usually resolve the problem.

Old-fashioned remedies

- **Arnica** – Using a few drops of arnica in warm water rinse the mouth with the solution as needed, then spit out, do not swallow
- **Basil** – Make a decoction of basil leaves by mashing the leaves and then boiling these in water. Ginger and honey can be added if desired. Allow to cool and then drink
- **Bay leaf** – Make a poultice of bay leaves after boiling these in water. When cool enough apply directly to the outside of the throat and leave for up to thirty minutes
- **Brown sugar** – Add to a mixture of warm water and lemon juice and drink or add between layers of sliced raw onions in a bowl then use the resulting juice as a cough medicine
- **Garlic** – Chew a clove of garlic each day until the sore throat has resolved
- **Ginger** – Finely grate fresh ginger into a cup and add boiling water, allow to cool to a comfortable temperature, then gargle and swallow. Honey and lemon juice can be added
- **Honey** – Eat a spoonful of honey. Alternatively, to warm water add a spoonful of honey and a squeeze of lemon juice, mix these together, then gargle or swallow
- **Lemon juice** – Mix one tablespoon of lemon juice in a cup of hot water, allow to cool to a comfortable temperature, then gargle and swallow. Honey can be added
- **Liquorice** – Mix powdered liquorice root with warm water, then gargle, and swallow
- **Peppermint** – Breath in the steam of hot water with peppermint oil added through the mouth taking care not to get too close to avoid the mouth getting burned
- **Salt** – Mix a third of a level teaspoon of salt into a cup of warm water and gargle. Do not swallow the mixture
- **Tea** – Add four to six tea bags to boiling water. Leave to steep for ten minutes, then

allow to cool to a comfortable temperature to enable the liquid to be gargled but not swallowed

- **Thyme** – Allow thyme tea to cool to a temperature that can be tolerated then gargle
- **Vinegar** – Mix one tablespoon of vinegar in warm water, gargle then swallow. Honey and lemon can be added
- **Witch hazel** – Boil a handful of leaves for around five minutes, strain, allow to cool to a tolerable temperature, and then gargle, spitting it out afterwards

SPLINTER

Getting a splinter of wood, or sometimes plastic, in the skin can be very painful. Moreover, the area may become infected, which is why it's best to remove the splinter.

Conventional treatment

After washing the hands thoroughly gently squeezing around the splinter helps it out, or exposes enough of the splinter so it can be removed by pulling it out with a clean pair of tweezers. Sometimes it's necessary to break the skin with a clean needle so the splinter can be grabbed. Once the splinter is removed the wound is washed, treated with antiseptic, and covered with a clean dressing or plaster.

Old-fashioned remedies

- **Epsom salts** – Soak the affected area in Epsom salts to aid removal of splinter
- **Oats** – Mix oatmeal, banana, and a tablespoon of water into a paste, apply to where the splinter is, leave for four to six hours to ease splinter removal
- **Radish** – Tape a slice of radish to the splintered and sore area, leave overnight, and the following morning swelling and splinter should be gone

STOMACH ULCER

The vast majority of stomach ulcers, also known as peptic ulcers, are caused by infection with the bacterium *Helicobacter pylori*. This infection damages the protective lining of the stomach and duodenum (upper part of the intestine) exposing the sensitive tissue underneath to powerful stomach acid, and this results in an ulcer forming. Most other peptic ulcers are due to side effects of anti-inflammatory painkillers that again upset the protective lining so acid is able to cause ulcers. Indigestion pain can be very severe, and if the ulcer perforates life-threatening haemorrhage may result.

Conventional treatment

Where infection is the cause this is usually treated with two antibiotics and a drug to reduce acid production. When anti-inflammatory medication is responsible if possible this is stopped and acid-reducing medication given whilst the ulcer heals.

Old-fashioned remedies

- **Cranberry** – Drink a glass of cranberry juice twice a day
- **Liquorice** – Take powdered liquorice in water or liquorice root tea once a day
- **Manuka honey** – Take a spoonful each day to help conventional treatment work

STRESS

Stress is a part of everyday life. Short-term bursts of stress keep us on our toes, out of danger, and help us to perform better at work and play. What we don't need is long-term stress that each day chips away at us and brings us down. This stress gives us stomach butterflies, a dry mouth, heart palpitations, and headaches amongst many other things. It also puts blood pressure up, makes it hard to concentrate, and leaves us feeling anxious and depressed. Relationship, financial, and work problems are often responsible, as are traffic congestion and interruptions when we don't want them.

Conventional treatment

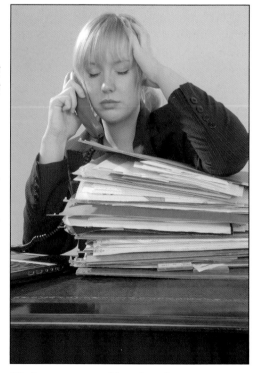

It's important to recognise the symptoms of stress – headaches, insomnia, a lack of energy or enthusiasm, for example, and avoid or remove any causes of stress. Have stress busters available to overcome stress when it comes your way, such as simple muscle stretches, herbal tea, deep breathing relaxation exercises, or favourite music, and take time to relax regularly so that stress isn't able to build up.

To prevent stress from building up it's important to eat regularly throughout the day, avoid drinking too much caffeine, get enough rest, and take regular time-outs to relax and unwind.

"Under pressure everything piles up"

Old-fashioned remedies

- **Bay leaf** – Place bay leaves, camomile, and bergamot into a cloth bag and rest head on this to help reduce stress
- **Camomile** – Drink a cup of camomile tea a few times a day. Alternatively, place a few drops of camomile essential oil onto clothing
- **Cloves** – Soak in a bath with added clove oil
- **Feverfew** – Drink an infusion of feverfew
- **Lavender** – Add essential oil to clothing, handkerchief, or a pillow. Inhale the steam from a hot lavender infusion, drink this, or add lavender to a warm bath and soak in this
- **Lemon balm** – Drink a warm lemon balm tea a couple of times a day
- **Lemon juice** – Place slices of fresh lemon in a hand towel soaked in warm water. Roll it up and warm in the microwave then put it loosely around the neck
- **Potato** – Make a potato poultice by boiling one or two large unpeeled potatoes until soft then mash. Remove excess moisture, wrap in a cloth, then place on the back of the neck

STRETCH MARKS

The more elastic the skin is, the greater the chances of developing stretch marks. Skin elasticity is often genetically determined, which is why stretch marks tend to run in families. The more the skin is stretched by pregnancy or weight gain, then the more likely stretch marks are to appear. It's difficult to prevent stretch marks since whether someone develops them or not is largely out of their control.

Conventional treatment

There are many creams and other skin treatments that claim to remove stretch marks. It's wise to try the less expensive ones since there is no real scientific evidence to say that any of these products actually work. Some people find that creams containing vitamin E and cocoa butter help. Cosmetic surgery and laser treatments can be used but can be uncomfortable and expensive, and may not always solve the problem. Fortunately, in time stretch marks will become paler, and much less noticeable.

Old-fashioned remedies

- **Aloe vera** – Apply fresh gel to the affected area and gently rub in
- **Coconut oil** – Rub in for three to four minutes a few times a day
- **Olive oil** – Rub in for three to four minutes a few times a day

STROKE

Most often the result of narrowed or furred up arteries caused by smoking, high cholesterol, and high blood pressure. This restricts blood flow and contributes to blood clots that prevent enough blood reaching the brain causing a mini-stroke, medically called a transient ischaemic attack (TIA), or blocking blood flow completely causing a stroke, sometimes called a 'brain attack'. Ruptured blood vessels causing a brain haemorrhage also cause strokes.

Conventional treatment

Don't smoke, and lose weight if needed. Exercise, a low fat diet, and minimal alcohol consumption helps to keep weight, blood pressure and cholesterol at healthy levels. Keep stress under control and eat oily fish each week. Medication is given to reduce the likelihood of blood clots forming and to keep blood pressure and cholesterol under control. Sometimes surgery is needed to widen the arteries or to remove blood clots from these.

Old-fashioned remedies

- **Bananas** – Eat one or two a day as they can help lower blood pressure
- **Garlic** – Consume up to three to four cloves a day. The allicin in garlic may help lower cholesterol and blood pressure
- **Oats** – Eat plenty as these help lower cholesterol
- **Omega-3** – Consume one to two portions of oily fish a week. Omega-3 essential fatty acids in these decrease the risk of blood clotting, irregular heart beats, and may lower blood pressure.

STYE

This infection of the root of an eyelash causes a swollen red lump on the edge of the eyelid. It's usually a bacterium called *Staphylococcus aureus* that naturally lives on the skin that's responsible for the infection.

Conventional treatment

Often there's no need for treatment as a stye will burst and heal on its own. A hot compress eases soreness and removes any pus. Sometimes antibiotic ointment is given.

Old-fashioned remedies

- **Camomile** – Brew a cup of camomile tea, remove tea bag and allow to cool until it's at a temperature that can be tolerated and rest against closed eyes

- **Cucumber** – Grate some cucumber and apply to the stye
- **Tea** – Wet a tea bag and place over the stye and leave for a few minutes

Sunburn

Excessive exposure to the sun damages the skin causing it to become red and tender. Sometimes the skin will blister. UV radiation and sunburn also increase the risk of skin cancer.

Sunburn is best avoided by staying in the shade between 11am and 3pm when the sun is most dangerous; covering up with loose baggy cotton clothes with sleeves and trouser legs, a legionnaire's cap or floppy hat with a wide brim, and sunglasses; and applying sunscreen of minimum SPF15 effective against UVA and UVB regularly throughout the day.

Conventional treatment

Get out of the sun and cool the skin by sponging with cool water. Painkillers and anti-inflammatory medication relieve pain, and sun cream or calamine lotion eases soreness and itching. It may be necessary to protect the burned area with a sterile dressing. Drinking water helps to rehydrate the skin. Keep an eye out for fever, rapid pulse, nausea and vomiting, or dizziness that may indicate heat exhaustion or heat stroke, which needs medical advice.

Old-fashioned remedies

- **Aloe vera** – Apply fresh gel to the affected area and gently rub in
- **Apples** – Cut an apple in half and then rub it against the skin
- **Bicarbonate of soda** – Mix bicarbonate of soda and water and apply to affected area
- **Calendula** – Apply as a tincture, poultice, compress, cream or ointment
- **Coconut oil** – Apply coconut oil to the affected area as required. Turmeric can be mixed with the coconut oil if desired
- **Cucumber** – Place a slice of cucumber against the sore skin or grind cucumber into a paste and then apply to sore area of skin
- **Frozen vegetables** – Place a bag of these wrapped in a cloth against the affected area
- **Ice** – Apply ice wrapped in cloth to the affected area
- **Oats** – Make an oatmeal paste by mixing uncooked oatmeal and water, and apply to the itchy areas either directly or by placing in muslin cloth
- **Potato** – Grate a potato and apply as a poultice
- **Tea** – Steep four tea bags in boiling water for ten minutes. Allow to cool, and then apply liquid to sunburned area using a cloth
- **Tomato** – Puree peeled tomatoes and add to a spoonful of yogurt or a spoonful of buttermilk and then apply to sunburn. Alternatively slice the tomatoes, dip in yogurt or buttermilk and apply to sunburn
- **Vinegar** – Mix two tablespoons of vinegar with a cup of water and apply to affected area

- **Yogurt** – Apply directly to affected area or soak in a cloth and dab onto the skin. Leave it to dry, and then rinse off with cool water

SWEATY FEET

Sweaty feet may not be a problem when they're hidden inside shoes and socks, but once released from these smelly feet can be very embarrassing. In fact, being kept in shoes and socks for long periods of time means sweat can't evaporate properly, allowing bacteria to digest the sweat and so produce the chemicals responsible for the characteristic smells. Under these warm and moist conditions fungi can also thrive and these too can produce an unpleasant smell.

Conventional treatment

The goal is to minimise how much sweat is available for bacteria to feed on. This is achieved by washing the feet regularly and drying them thoroughly; wearing clean socks each day as sweat accumulates on socks, and limiting how long feet are in sweat-encouraging closed footwear. Foot deodorants and antiperspirants or anti-fungal powders are sometimes recommended. Remove any dry skin as this allows bacteria to flourish.

Old-fashioned remedies

- **Bicarbonate of soda** – Powder onto the feet each day
- **Epsom salts** – Add one or two tablespoons of Epsom salts to a bowl of warm water and then allow the feet to soak for ten to fifteen minutes
- **Oats** – Place oatmeal in the socks

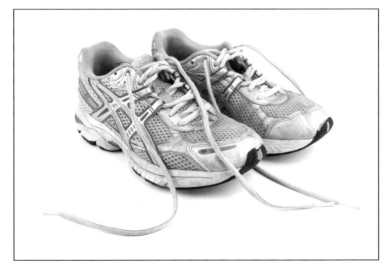

"Everything deserves a break"

- **Radish** – After bathing or showering pat feet dry, and then apply a handful of radish juice onto the feet and in between the toes as necessary

Thrush

Thrush is a yeast infection caused by a fungus called *Candida albicans* that naturally lives in the vagina and the genital area. In women it can cause vulval itching, irritation, soreness, vaginal discharge, and pain when urinating and during sex. In men it can cause redness, soreness, and itching of the penis. When someone is run down, has been taking antibiotics, or is pregnant they are more likely to develop thrush infection. Uncontrolled or undiagnosed diabetes can result in repeated thrush infections.

Conventional treatment

Wearing cotton underwear, not wearing tight clothes, using sanitary towels rather than tampons and not using perfumed soaps is often advised. Try using aqueous cream instead of usual soap or shower gel and resist the urge to be overhygienic since washing too often can promote thrush. Thrush is treated with anti-fungal cream, vaginal pessaries, or capsules. Sometimes sexual partners are advised to be treated at the same time.

Old-fashioned remedies

- **Aloe vera** – Apply fresh gel externally to the affected area and gently rub in
- **Calendula** – Apply externally as a tincture, poultice, compress, cream or ointment
- **Cucumber** – Place a slice of cucumber against the sore skin or grind cucumber into a paste and then apply to sore area of skin
- **Garlic** – Crush garlic and apply externally to the affected area
- **Tomato** – Puree peeled tomatoes and add to a spoonful of yogurt or a spoonful of buttermilk and then apply externally. Alternatively slice the tomatoes, dip in yogurt or buttermilk and apply externally to affected areas
- **Yogurt** – Put plain live yogurt into the vagina using a tampon applicator

Tired eyes

Tired eyes can indicate that it's time for an eye test and that glasses, contact lenses, or a new prescription if someone's already using these, are necessary. Tired eyes may simply be because someone is generally tired, or that they are stressed. Stress often causes the muscles around the eyes to feel tight or twitch. Spending long periods of time looking at a computer, or if the screen is too bright, causes eye-strain and makes the eyes feel tired. Eyes can feel tired if they've been exposed to too much UV light.

Conventional treatment

The eyes need rest too so whether it's time spent in front of a computer screen or close work give them a break every fifteen to twenty minutes. Protect them from UV light with sunglasses, and have an eye test. Relaxing often relieves tired eyes as does bathing them.

Old-fashioned remedies

- **Camomile** – Brew a cup of camomile tea, remove the tea bag and allow to cool until it's at a temperature that can be tolerated and rest it against closed eyes
- **Cucumber** – Place a chilled slice of cucumber over the closed eyelids
- **Papaya** – Make a poultice of mashed papaya fruit and place over closed eyes
- **Potato** – Extract juice from one or two potatoes, soak cotton wool in the juice, and gently hold against closed eyes
- **Tea** – Add a tea bag to boiled water, leave for around five minutes and then remove, squeeze out and allow to cool to a tolerable temperature then place over closed eyes
- **Thyme** – Make a compress of thyme tea and place gently over closed eyes

TIREDNESS

There are many causes of tiredness. Physical ones include anaemia, diabetes, an under-active thyroid, and the side effects of medication. Stress, anxiety, and depression are emotional causes, and overdoing it at work or socially are very common reasons why someone may feel tired some or all of the time. A lack of a good night's sleep is often the reason.

Tiredness not only affects performance, it also affects concentration, makes accidents more likely, and leaves someone susceptible to infections.

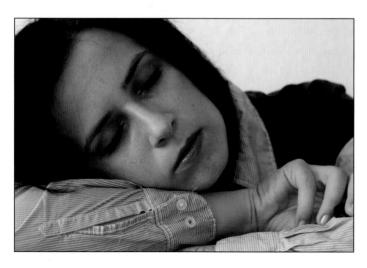

"Fit to drop"

Conventional treatment

This depends on the underlying cause. If iron deficiency is responsible, for example, extra iron solves the problem. If depression is the reason treating this eliminates feelings of tiredness. Focussing on boosting energy with exercise, energy-rich foods, B vitamins and relaxation helps, as does taking regular time-outs and reducing alcohol consumption.

Old-fashioned remedies

- **Camomile** – Drink a cup of camomile tea to relax the mind and body
- **Lavender** – Drink a relaxing lavender infusion
- **Tea** – Drink a cup of black tea, it's a natural pick-me-up

TOOTHACHE

Toothache usually occurs when a nerve in the tooth is irritated but can also occur as a consequence of tooth decay or infection. Bacteria in the mouth feed on food debris and sugar and whilst doing this produce the acid responsible for dental decay. Other problems that may contribute to toothache are plaque and inflamed, swollen, and painful gums – all indicators of inadequate dental hygiene.

Conventional treatment

With good dental care and hygiene dental problems and toothache can be prevented. Brushing and flossing removes food and sugar left in the mouth reducing the risk of acid production and plaque build-up that damages the teeth and gums. A mouthwash can help to reduce gum inflammation. It's important to keep consumption of sugary foods and drinks to a minimum. Regular dental check-ups help to identify problems earlier rather than later. Painkillers and anti-inflammatory drugs relieve pain.

Old-fashioned remedies

- **Camomile** – Allow a cup of camomile herb tea to cool and then use as a mouth rinse
- **Cloves** – Chew a clove and roll it

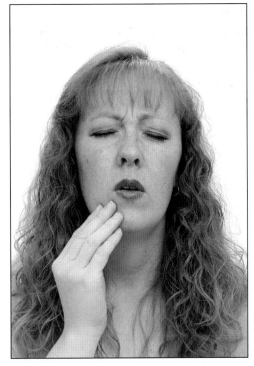

"Ouch, that hurts"

around the sore part of the mouth or dip a cotton bud in clove oil and apply directly to
the sore area

- **Horseradish** – Grate horseradish and apply to the gums near to the aching tooth
- **Ice** – Suck and roll an ice cube around the mouth
- **Lemon juice** – Apply lemon juice to the painful area
- **Thyme** – Make a cup of thyme tea by infusing a sprig of thyme in hot water, and once
  cool enough rinse around the mouth

TRAVEL SICKNESS

This occurs when the brain receives mixed and inconsistent messages from the eyes and
balance mechanisms in the ear about the body's position. The result, feelings of nausea,
sweating, vomiting, and a bad start to a day out or holiday. Smells, food, and keeping the
head down focussing on books when travelling, for example, can set things off.

Conventional treatment

Anti-sickness medication and acupressure wrist bands are popular. In a car have a clear view
of the road ahead and avoid too much time looking down towards your lap. The car should
be well ventilated and the driver shouldn't take bends too quickly or repeatedly accelerate
and slow down. On board a boat keep away from fuel fumes and food, keep on deck
focussing on something on the horizon, and if inside keep to the middle of the vessel on as
lower deck as possible. In flight try and sit near the wing because the plane is most stable
here. Keeping eyes closed helps.

Old-fashioned remedies

- **Basil** – Make an infusion of basil in boiling water, allow to cool, and then drink
- **Cloves** – Chew on one or two cloves and then spit these out
- **Ginger** – Eat fresh, crystallised, in biscuits or drink ginger tea
- **Lavender** – Drink a cup of lavender tea
- **Onions** – Place a slice of raw onion under each armpit
- **Peppermint** – Drink peppermint tea

VARICOSE VEINS

Inside veins are valves that prevent the blood from flowing in the wrong direction. Being
overweight, standing for long periods of time, having to strain on the toilet because of constipation all put extra pressure on the valves in the veins, making them incompetent so they
don't work as well as they should. The veins then become swollen and very visible, called
varicose veins.

Not only do the veins become visibly swollen and distorted, the legs may ache, feel heavy, and be uncomfortable. When severe the skin over the vein can become dry, itchy, and thin, and an ulcer may develop.

Conventional treatment.

It's important to avoid anything that puts extra pressure on the veins, for instance straining on the toilet. Regular exercise helps prevent varicose veins from developing or getting worse. Elastic support stockings and cream or supplements containing extract of horse chestnut can help lessen the size and appearance of varicose veins.

Injecting chemicals into the veins, called sclerotherapy, closes off the veins, or surgically removing the veins is often undertaken.

Old-fashioned remedies

- **Aloe vera** – Apply fresh gel to the affected area and gently rub in
- **Calendula** – Drink calendula tea, made by infusing the petals, twice daily
- **Witch hazel** – Apply witch hazel cream or tincture to the varicose veins

WARTS AND VERRUCAS

Warts are caused by infection with different strains of the human papilloma virus (HPV) that causes rough skin-coloured small lumps to appear on the skin. Most often they appear on the hands and fingers, but can appear anywhere on the body. On the feet they are called verrucas. Warts may look unsightly but generally they don't cause any problems, although verrucas may hurt. These viruses are very contagious and are passed on through close skin-to-skin contact, particularly if the skin is damaged or wet. For example, verrucas are easily caught at public swimming pools.

Conventional treatment

Within a few years most warts and verrucas will have cleared up without needing treatment, but treatment helps get rid of them more quickly. Creams, gels and paints are used, as is freezing with liquid nitrogen therapy. Sometimes surgery and laser treatment is used to treat more stubborn warts and verrucas.

Old-fashioned remedies

- **Banana** – Cut a piece of banana skin large enough to cover the wart or verruca, tape it securely in place (inner side of the peel against the verruca or wart) and leave overnight repeating each night until the verruca or wart disappears
- **Calendula** – Apply as a tincture on cotton wool to the wart or verruca
- **Carrots** – Mix olive oil with grated carrot and apply the mixture to the wart or verruca

directly or using a clean cloth. Hold in place with a clean dressing for up to an hour or overnight. Repeat this daily until wart or verruca has gone

- **Coconut oil** – Rub coconut oil directly onto the wart or verruca, and repeat this each day until cleared. Alternatively apply coconut oil to the pad of a sticking plaster, place this over the wart or verruca and leave overnight
- **Figs** – Press half a freshly sliced fig against the wart or verruca and fix in place overnight. The fig can also be mashed so it becomes mushy and applied to the wart or verruca
- **Lemon juice** – Place a slice of lemon over the wart or verruca and keep it in place with tape and leave overnight. Repeat this daily until wart or verruca has gone
- **Onions** – After applying fresh lemon juice to the wart or verruca place raw chopped onion onto the wart. Leave for ten to twenty minutes. Repeat two to three times daily
- **Papaya** – Drip the milky latex from a green papaya onto the wart or verruca two to three times daily until cleared
- **Potato** – Slice a potato in half and rub the flesh against the wart or verruca, or cut a slice of potato and tape this against the wart overnight repeating daily until wart disappears
- **Tea** – Moisten a tea bag and then tape against the wart or verruca. Leave in place for thirty to sixty minutes

WAXY EARS

The ear makes wax as part of its self-cleaning mechanism. Sometimes this builds up and can cause the ear to feel blocked and sounds to be dull or quieter than usual. One of the commonest causes of wax build up is using cotton wool buds to try and clean the ear. Doing this compacts wax and pushes it further into the ear making it harder for it to come out of the ear, as left alone it would do naturally. Sometimes this wax build up can feel uncomfortable.

Conventional treatment

Don't put anything smaller than your elbow into your ear, is the simplest advice to prevent wax build up. When waxy ears are causing a problem softening drops can be used to soften wax, which then if necessary can be removed by syringing the ears.

Old-fashioned remedies

- **Bicarbonate of soda** – Dissolve bicarbonate of soda in water and add three to four drops to each ear
- **Olive oil** – Add three to four drops of olive oil to the ear from a teaspoon or with a dropper
- **Salt** – Add salt to warm water and gently irrigate the ear canal using a dropper or a teaspoon

WIND

It's a normal part of digestion for bacteria and enzymes to break down food in the gut. This process results in gas being produced and it's a fact of life that some people naturally produce more gas than others. Gas produced in the upper gut comes out as a burp, and that produced in the lower part as wind. In fact, it's thought to be normal to pass wind up to thirty times a day.

High-fibre foods, spicy foods, Brussels sprouts, cabbage, pulses and beer cause lots of gas to be produced. Some medical conditions are associated with excess passage of wind, such as irritable bowel syndrome (IBS), lactose intolerance, and constipation.

Conventional treatment

Reducing consumption of these foods, eating more slowly and chewing food more, and not gulping down drinks helps reduce the amount of air swallowed into the gut and overall gas amounts so there's less to come out. Exercise helps to disperse gas, probiotics are thought to be of assistance, and remedies are available to help control excess wind.

Old-fashioned remedies

- **Bay leaf** – Make an infusion of bay leaves and drink once or twice a day
- **Camomile** – Drink a cup of camomile tea once or twice a day
- **Lavender** – Drink a cup of lavender tea a couple of times a day
- **Liquorice** – Chew and swallow liquorice or mix half a teaspoon of liquorice root powder with warm water and drink. Liquorice tea can also be used
- **Peppermint** – Drink one or two cups of peppermint tea immediately after eating
- **Thyme** – Drink one or two cups of thyme tea immediately after eating

Index

Aching feet 65, 87, 92, 100, 157–8

Aching joints 109, 121

Aching muscles 50, 71

Acne 11, 23, 65, 87, 130

Alcohol 10, 112, 114, 119, 122, 129, 133, 138, 152, 157–8, 161, 164, 166, 169, 173–4, 181–2, 188, 194, 199

Alertness 105

Allicin 61–3, 139, 164–5, 185, 194

Allyl isothiocyanate 64, 96

Almond oil 47, 117

Aloe Vera 4–6, 143, 146–7, 154, 156, 160, 167, 169, 178, 183–4, 186–7, 193, 195, 197, 201

Alzheimer's disease 116, 131

Anaesthetic 40–1, 64, 90, 132, 176

Anal fissure 131–2

Analgesic 40

Ankle 59–60, 67, 69, 169

Ankle sprain 60, 69

Anti-allergy 80, 103

Antibacterial 17, 31–2, 62, 64–5, 89, 120

Anti-fungal 10–11, 31–2, 43–4, 120, 126, 135, 152, 187, 196, 197

Antihistamine 8, 86, 162

Anti-inflammatory 10–11, 17, 29–35, 43, 53–4, 71, 80, 86, 89, 103, 115–8, 123, 133, 140, 142–3, 149, 159, 166, 170–1, 174, 177, 182, 190–2

Anti-microbial 10–11, 34

Antiseptic 31–3, 35, 40–1, 71, 90, 108–10, 120, 129, 151, 191

Anti-spasmodic 33–4

Antiviral 17, 31–2, 62, 73–4, 144, 146

Anxiety 34–5, 54, 70, 73, 80, 86, 132, 138, 153, 168, 179, 181, 190, 198

Aphrodisiac 38, 65, 85, 88, 111

Apple 6–9, 24–5, 34, 40–1, 56, 86, 112, 119, 120–1, 134, 140, 149, 154, 156, 162, 167, 183–4, 187, 195

Arnica 9–12, 60, 130, 133, 135–6, 140, 142, 159–60, 170, 177, 180, 190

Arsenic 127

Artery 76, 82, 138, 164–5, 172, 194

Arthritis 17, 20, 53, 57, 60, 65, 111, 115–6, 129, 133, 157–8, 169–70, 184

Asthma 79, 128, 134

Athlete's foot 11, 40, 44, 63, 108–9, 120, 126, 135, 158

Back pain 65, 101, 135–6

Bad breath 41, 73–4, 80, 97, 112, 125, 136–7

Baking soda 22, 117, 119

Banana 9, 12–5, 84, 139, 142, 147, 154, 161, 163–7, 174–5, 191, 194, 201

Basil 15–8, 133, 136, 138, 149, 159, 168, 170–1, 176–7, 179, 190, 200

Bay Leaf 18–21, 133, 136, 141, 152, 159, 169–70, 172, 177, 190, 193, 203

Belch see Excess Wind

Bicarbonate of soda 21–4, 77, 130, 140, 145, 152, 154, 156, 166, 168, 183, 187, 195–6, 202

Bites 14, 22, 48, 71, 77, 98, 106, 117, 167

Blackheads 52, 77, 130

Bladder 47, 49, 151

Bleeding 26, 59, 60, 68, 77, 106, 118, 122–3, 151, 180

Blemish 77

Blisters 38–9, 137, 144, 146, 166, 195

Bloating 17, 80, 91, 138, 146–7, 169, 182

Blocked ears 104, 202

Blocked nose 6, 91, 97, 148, 161, 178

Blood pressure 13, 48, 50, 61, 63, 81, 101, 104, 128, 138–9, 164–5, 172, 194

Body odour 23, 98, 120, 139, 140

Boils 10, 29, 46, 57, 65, 77, 87, 109

Bones 16, 86, 124

Bowel 4–6, 9, 12, 30, 35, 37, 49, 55–7, 74, 80, 82, 91, 93, 125, 138, 146–7, 153, 160, 169, 203

Breast tenderness 60, 140, 182

Breath freshener 92

Bronchitis 79, 141

Brown sugar 24–7, 135, 142–3, 147, 149, 151, 154, 165, 181, 190

Bruise 10–11, 14, 26, 59, 87, 95, 98, 120–3, 142

Burns 5, 26, 31–2, 38, 71, 87, 89, 97, 109, 121, 126, 137, 143, 185

Cabbage 27–30, 100, 133, 136, 140–1, 147, 159, 181–2, 203

Calendula 30–3, 132, 135, 143, 146, 154, 156, 160, 166, 168, 180, 187, 195, 197, 201

Callus 31, 46, 87, 106, 121, 147–8, 158

Calmative 33–4, 90, 92

Camomile 20, 33–6, 53, 133, 157, 162–3, 168–9, 173, 176, 181, 183, 189, 193–4, 198–9, 203

Cancer 7, 28, 31, 45, 76, 82, 86, 105, 111, 116, 128, 195

Carrots 36–9, 58, 96, 137, 143, 145, 154, 156, 183–4, 187, 201

Cellulite 89, 100

Chapped lips 47, 106, 144

Chapped skin 84

Chest 11, 20, 66, 74, 141, 149

Chewing gum 119

Chickenpox 23, 84, 117, 137, 144

Chilblains 87, 104, 145

Chills 34

Cholesterol 7, 28, 45, 48, 61, 63, 76, 82, 86, 164–5, 172, 194

Circles under eyes 95

Circulation 7, 10–11, 16, 28, 31, 45, 48, 62–3, 71, 76, 81, 86, 105, 165, 185

Clove oil 40–1, 132, 154, 160, 193, 200

Cloves 39–41, 61–3, 132, 137, 139, 149, 154, 160–1, 164–5, 179, 185–6, 193–4, 199–200

Coconut 7, 41–4, 117, 130–1, 145, 152, 154–6, 183–4, 187–8, 193, 195, 202

Coconut oil 41–4, 117, 130–1, 145, 152, 154–6, 183–4, 187–8, 193, 195, 202

Cold sores 6, 32, 68, 73–4, 107, 123, 146

Colds 17, 26, 62, 63, 109, 112, 115, 148, 190

Colicky abdominal pain 54, 129

Compress 10–11, 17, 29, 32–3, 54, 60, 71, 74, 109, 120, 13–4, 140, 142–3, 146, 151, 154, 156–7, 159–60, 166–8, 17–1, 177–8, 180, 187, 189, 19–5, 197–8

Concentration 24, 85, 105, 198

Congestion 6, 65–6, 74, 92, 97, 103, 149, 162, 178, 188, 192

Constipation 6, 12, 14, 26, 29, 49, 51, 55, 80, 82, 84, 89, 127, 131, 138, 146–7, 160, 169, 200, 203

Cooling 29, 49, 69, 74, 90, 92, 107, 144

Corns 31, 46, 77, 83, 87, 89, 106, 121, 147–8, 158

Cough 9, 17, 26, 41, 62–3, 65, 80–1, 92, 109, 112, 115, 134, 135, 141, 146, 148, 149, 150, 171, 178, 190

Cradle cap 150

Cramps 26, 54, 80, 114–5, 146, 172, 181–2

Cranberry 44–7, 144, 148, 152, 160, 192

Croup 150

Cucumber 47–50, 126, 130, 139, 147, 154, 156–7, 183–4, 186–7, 189, 195, 197, 198

Curcumin 116

Cut 4, 8, 9, 14–5, 26 29, 38, 62, 71 77, 87, 95, 98, 102, 122–3, 143, 145, 151, 154, 156, 167–8, 176, 183–4, 187, 195, 201–2

Cystitis 4–5, 22, 47, 103, 151–2

Dandruff 20, 43, 77, 120, 152, 187

Decongestant 90, 92, 148, 178

Depression 73–4, 86, 127, 131, 153, 168, 173, 180–1, 198–9

Dermatitis 31, 43, 49, 71, 80, 150, 155, 186

Diarrhoea 9, 11, 12, 26, 40, 153–4, 169, 179

Dry skin 6, 38, 44, 126, 154, 196

Earache 104, 117

Earwax 22, 104, 202

Eczema 33, 84, 117, 121, 154–5, 186–7

Energy 7, 12, 42, 65, 81–2, 84, 93, 107, 146, 173, 192, 199

Epsom salts 50–2, 141–2, 147, 158, 177, 191, 196

Excess wind 146, 203

Exfoliant 26, 38, 51, 89

Expectorant 65–6, 81

Eye 8, 36, 42, 47–9, 52, 59, 64, 69, 84–5, 87–9, 95–6, 106, 109–10, 128, 156–7, 161–2, 189, 194–5, 197–8, 200

Face scrub 126

Fever 52, 54, 109, 114–5, 144, 149–50, 157, 190, 195

Feverfew 52–5, 133–4, 157, 159, 163, 170, 172, 174, 177, 180–1, 183, 193

Fibre 7, 9, 12, 28–9, 37, 40, 43, 45, 48–9, 56, 82, 84, 86, 93, 105, 111, 132, 138, 146–7, 154, 160, 169, 203

Figs 55, 56–8, 134, 159, 170, 177, 202

Flaky skin 66

Flatulence 28

Fluid retention 49, 138, 182

Folic acid 7, 86, 97

Foot odour 51, 106

Formaldehyde 128

Freckles 47, 77

Freshener 36, 80, 92

Frozen vegetables 58–61, 67, 134, 141–2, 151, 154, 156, 159–60, 163, 170, 174, 177, 180, 188, 195

Garlic 61–3, 102, 135, 137, 139, 146, 149, 164–5, 172, 178, 185–6, 190, 194, 197

Genitals 103, 117, 139–40197

Gin 113–5, 129

Ginger 17, 26, 40, 116, 134, 138–9, 149, 161, 163, 171–9, 181–3, 185, 190, 200

Glycyrrhizin 79–80

Gout 29, 60, 133, 158–9, 169

Graze 151

Gum disease 45, 105, 136

Gut spasm 35, 80, 169

Haemorrhoids 5, 32, 41, 46, 55, 68, 87, 118, 121, 123, 160–1

Hair 5, 20, 27, 31, 34, 38, 40, 43, 49–50, 52, 77, 120, 130, 134, 150, 152, 155, 182, 185–7

Halitosis 112, 136

Hangover 14, 41, 78, 112, 161–2, 179

Hayfever 8, 36, 120, 161–2, 178, 189

Headache 14, 29, 52, 54–5, 60, 65–6, 68, 70–1, 81, 86, 92, 95, 127–8, 161–3, 173–4, 192

Heart attack 48, 50, 61, 63, 82–3, 104, 138, 164–5

Heart disease 7, 83, 111, 164

Heartburn 8, 14, 22, 166

Herpes 74, 103, 117, 137, 146

Hiccups 26, 68, 164, 165

High blood pressure 13, 48, 61, 101, 138, 164, 194

Honey 9, 17, 47, 49, 62, 65–6, 70, 73, 77, 87, 91, 117, 120, 130–2, 134, 137, 143, 149, 151, 155, 156, 160, 162, 166, 171–2, 176, 183, 188, 190, 191–2

Horseradish 63–6, 96, 130, 134, 136, 149, 155, 156, 158–9, 163, 168, 171, 174, 177, 179, 183, 188, 200

Hydrogen sulphide 61, 126

Ice 12, 58–60, 66–70, 73, 97, 100, 116, 134, 137, 142–4, 146, 151, 155–7, 159–60, 163, 165, 168, 170–1, 174, 176–7, 180, 183–4, 186, 188, 195, 200

Impetigo 32, 165–6

Indigestion 14, 22, 40, 71, 74, 80, 89, 91, 161, 166, 191

Inflammation 14–5, 17, 29, 31, 52, 58, 65, 69, 71, 95, 104, 116–7, 123, 130, 133, 151, 157–8, 166, 170–2, 177–8, 199

Inflammatory bowel disease 4

Inhalation 178

Insect bite 14, 22, 71, 98, 167

Insect repellent 34, 53, 73, 110, 167

Insect stings 77

Insoluble fibre 82, 84

Insomnia 34, 35, 71, 168, 192

Irritable bowel syndrome 4, 6, 35, 80, 82, 91, 138, 147, 169, 203

Irritated skin 4, 5, 8, 12, 23, 35, 49, 54, 77, 120, 167, 187

Irritation 22, 128, 151, 154, 166, 197

Itchy ears 121, 161

Itchy skin 38, 66, 84, 117, 120–1, 123

Joint pain 104, 116–7

Laryngitis 79, 171

Lavender 69–72, 131–4, 143, 151, 159, 163, 166, 168–9, 171, 173–5, 177, 179, 181–183, 193, 199, 200, 203

Laxative 5, 49, 50, 80, 127, 132, 147

Leg cramps 114–5, 172

Lemon 8, 26, 57, 62, 72–8, 87, 114–5, 117–8, 120, 130–1, 133–5, 137, 141, 144, 146, 148–9, 151–3, 159–60, 166, 168, 171–2, 178–81, 186–7, 190–1, 193, 200, 202

Lemon balm 72–5, 131, 134, 137, 141, 144, 146, 153, 159, 166, 171, 178, 179, 181, 193

Lemon juice 8, 75–8, 87, 114, 130, 135, 148–9, 151–2, 168, 172, 180, 187, 190, 193, 200, 202

Libido 86, 173

Liquorice 78–81, 135, 137–8, 141, 147, 149, 167, 169, 172, 176, 183, 190, 192, 203

Longevity 73–4

Malaria 114

Marigolds 30, 32–3

Mastitis 28–9, 100, 140

Meditation 34

Melissa 73

Memory 69, 73, 87, 131

Menstrual 26, 54, 80, 146, 174, 181–2

Menstrual cramps 26, 80

Mercury 127, 128

Migraine vii, 52–5, 173–4

Milk 28, 42, 65, 105, 122, 124–5, 134, 136, 140, 145, 155–6, 159, 161, 169, 171, 177, 183, 188

Moisturiser 26, 38, 126

Molasses 24–7, 142

Mood–lifting 36

Morning sickness 15, 175, 179

Motion sickness 17

Mouth freshener 80

Mouth ulcers 6, 11, 17, 35, 55, 80, 103, 107, 175–6

Mouthwash 10, 38, 41, 46, 109, 176, 199

Muscle 10–11, 16, 20, 33, 50–1, 65, 69–71, 73, 86, 91–2, 101, 109, 114–5, 117, 122, 135, 162, 164, 170, 172, 176–8, 192, 197

Muscle relaxing 33

Muscle tension 70

Nasal congestion 92, 103, 149, 162, 178

Nausea 17, 41, 55, 71, 78, 87, 92, 146, 161, 174–5, 179, 195, 200

Nervousness 70

Neuralgia 95, 179–80

Night cramps 115

Nosebleed 60, 77, 180

Oatmeal 81–4, 126, 145, 148, 155–6, 158, 168–9, 184, 188, 191, 195–6

Oats 81–3, 147–8, 158, 164–5, 191, 194–6

Odour 23, 51, 53, 61, 98, 106, 112, 120, 126, 136, 139–40

Olive oil 20, 38–9, 49, 51, 92, 133, 136–7, 139, 145, 147, 150, 155–6, 158–9, 161, 170, 177, 184, 187–8, 193, 201–2

Onion 26, 40, 61, 84–7, 131, 135, 137, 142–3, 145, 148–9, 153, 160, 163, 173–5, 179, 183, 190–200, 202

Painful joints 60, 66, 117, 170

Painful periods 53, 54, 181

Painkillers 26, 55, 132–3, 136, 141–3, 146, 148, 151–2, 159, 161–2, 167, 170–1, 174, 177–8, 180–1, 190–1, 195, 199

Palpitations 70, 133, 181, 192

Papain 88–90

Papaya 87–90, 131, 143, 147, 148, 157, 167, 186, 189, 198, 202

Parsley 87, 107

Pawpaw 87–8

Peas 58–60, 79, 141

Pectin 7, 9

Peppermint 90–2, 138, 142, 148–9, 158, 161, 167, 169, 172, 175, 178–9, 189–90, 200, 203

Peptic ulcer 29, 191

Period pain 181

Period cramps *see* Painful periods

Periods 46, 181, 184, 196–7, 200

Piles 46, 60, 95, 160, 192

Pimples 33, 43, 49, 103, 117

Porridge 81–4, 147

Potassium 7, 13, 16, 37, 48, 56, 64, 86, 88, 93, 97, 152

Potato 93–6, 134, 141–2, 155–7, 159–60, 163, 171, 175, 178, 180, 184–5, 188–9, 193, 195, 198, 202

Poultice 8, 10–11, 14, 20, 32–3, 38, 46, 54, 57, 80, 86–7, 89, 95, 104, 132–4, 136, 140–3, 146, 148, 154–7, 159–60, 163, 168, 170, 172, 174–5, 177, 180, 184, 187–90, 193, 195, 197–8

Pregnancy 2, 15, 43, 48, 50, 140, 147, 160, 166, 175, 179, 193, 197

Premenstrual syndrome (PMS) 43, 80, 86, 182–3

Prickly heat 183

Probiotic 169

Prostate cancer 28, 111

Psoriasis 84, 102, 117, 154, 184, 187

Puffy eyes 36, 106

Quinine 113–5, 149, 172

Radish 65, 96–8, 140, 142–3, 168, 179, 191, 197
Raynaud's phenomenon 93, 185
Razor burn 126, 185
Reflux 8, 166, 190
Relax 35, 51, 69–71, 73–4, 91–2, 103, 109, 119, 142, 152, 177, 192, 199
RICE technique 170, 177
Ringworm 40, 117, 186
Rolling pin 29–30, 48, 98–101, 136, 141, 158, 189
Rough skin 26, 52, 201

Saffron 32, 117
Sagging skin 97
Salt 50–2, 63, 87, 93, 95, 96, 101–4, 118–9, 131, 138–9, 141–2, 145, 147, 152, 155–6, 158, 172, 176–7, 179, 182–4, 188, 190–1, 196, 202
Scaly skin 95
Scar 5, 44, 151
Scurvy 28, 29, 46, 76
Sea air 103
Seborrhoeic 150, 155, 186
Selenium 82
Serotonin 12, 48, 52
Shaving nicks 68, 123
Sickness 15, 17, 92, 174–5, 179, 200
Sinus congestion 65
Sitz baths 54
Skin irritation 5, 8, 12, 23, 35, 49, 54, 77, 187
Skin toning 49
Skin ulcers 89
Sleep 20, 34–5, 71, 109, 115, 153, 156–7, 168–9, 172, 188–9, 198
Smelly feet 196
Snoring 100, 178, 188
Sodium bicarbonate 21
Soluble fibre 7, 82

Sore breasts 95, 100, 141
Sore eyes 36, 49, 89, 95, 109, 189
Sore feet 44, 77, 91
Sore gums 17, 109
Sore joints 54, 60, 95, 104, 171
Sore muscles 20, 51, 57, 71, 92, 122, 177
Sore skin 6, 14, 43, 49, 92, 95, 154, 156, 183–4, 186–7, 195, 197
Sore throat 17, 20, 26, 75, 77, 80–1, 103, 107, 109, 118, 120, 123, 141, 148, 149, 171–2, 190
Sores 6, 32, 38, 57, 68, 71, 73, 74, 75, 89, 107, 117, 123, 146, 186
Spasm 34, 35, 52, 80, 114–5, 169, 172, 179
Splinter 52, 84, 97, 191
Spots 11, 77, 87, 89, 109, 130–1, 144
Sprains 11, 60, 69, 170
Steak 59
Steam 6, 9, 71, 92, 122, 131, 133–4, 143, 149–50, 162–3, 169, 172–4, 178–9, 181–3, 189–90, 193
Stiffness 11, 133
Sting 14, 17, 22, 31, 66, 77, 98, 106, 117, 120, 167–8, 185
Stomach ulcers 45, 80, 166, 191
Strain 69, 146, 162, 176, 189, 197, 200–1
Stress 20, 33–4, 36, 41, 54, 71, 74, 77, 93, 100, 130–1, 133, 137–8, 146–7, 152, 154–5, 158, 162–4, 166, 169, 173–4, 176–7, 179, 185, 187, 192–4, 197–8
Stretch marks 44, 193
Stroke 13, 48, 50, 61, 63, 82, 83, 104, 138, 165, 194–5
Stye 106, 194–5
Sugar 14–5, 24–7, 42, 70, 79, 82, 100, 124, 135, 142–3, 147, 149, 151–2, 154, 161, 165, 181, 190, 199
Sunburn 4, 23, 32, 43, 49, 68, 84, 95, 106, 112, 120, 126, 195
Sweaty feet 82, 196
Sweeten 56, 77, 124

Swelling 11, 14, 29, 49, 58–60, 68–9, 95, 97, 103, 133, 140, 158–9, 167, 170, 177–8, 188, 191
Swollen joints 54, 67, 74

Tea 11, 20, 26, 31–6, 47, 54, 60, 71, 73–4, 78–80, 91–2, 100, 104–7, 109–10, 123, 131–5, 137–8, 141–5, 147–9, 152–3, 155–9, 161–3, 166–83, 185–6, 188–95, 198–203
Tea bags 104–7, 145, 148, 155–7, 162, 168, 176, 188–90, 194–5, 198, 202
Teeth 9, 38, 40, 66, 77, 89, 105, 124, 136, 175, 199, 200
Thrush 124, 126, 197
Thyme 107–10, 131, 134–5, 143, 149, 157–9, 171, 178, 189, 191, 198, 200, 203
Thymol 108
Thyroid gland 28, 173, 181
Tired eyes 48, 197, 198
Tired feet 29, 52, 92, 112
Tiredness 57, 115, 168, 173, 174, 188, 197–9
Tomato 15, 110, 111–3, 137, 155–6, 158, 161, 188, 195, 197
Tonic water 113–5, 149, 157, 172
Toning 49
Tooth decay 105, 136, 199
Toothache 40–1, 66, 68, 77, 109, 127, 199
Travel sickness 200
Turmeric 43, 115–8, 130–1, 134, 145, 151, 154–6, 159–60, 171, 178, 184, 186–8, 195
Twisted 59, 67, 169

Ulcerative colitis 4, 153
Ulcers 6, 11, 17, 29, 35, 45, 55, 80, 89, 103, 107, 166, 175–6, 191

Upset stomach 15, 20, 89

Varicose veins 32, 121–2, 160, 200–1
Varicosities 95
Vegetables 9, 28, 37, 58–61, 67, 86, 94, 97, 102, 111, 134, 141–2, 151, 154, 156, 159–60, 163, 170, 174, 177, 180, 188, 195
Verruca 15, 44, 89, 158, 201–2
Vinegar 85, 93, 100, 103–4, 118–21, 127, 131, 134, 140, 142, 145, 148, 152, 155–6, 159, 162, 168, 171–2, 178, 186–8, 191, 195
Vomiting 11, 87, 127, 161, 174–5, 179, 195, 200
Vulval varicosities 95

Warts 15, 31, 38, 44, 57, 77, 87, 89, 95, 106, 128, 201–2
Water 5–6, 10, 11, 17, 20, 22–3, 25–6, 29, 35, 38, 42, 44, 45, 47–9, 51–2, 57, 59, 60, 62, 64, 66–8, 72–4, 76–85, 87, 89, 92, 97, 100–7, 109, 113–5, 117–23, 126, 130–8, 140–9, 151–2, 154–72, 174, 176–9, 181–4, 186–93, 195–96, 198, 200, 202–3
Wax 22, 104, 202
Waxy ears see Ear wax
Weeping sores 89
Wind 20, 27, 71, 80, 91–3, 138, 144, 146, 154, 169, 203
Witch hazel 60, 121–3, 132, 142, 145–6, 151, 155–6, 161, 178, 180, 186, 188, 191,
Wound 4–5, 10, 17, 26, 31, 46, 57, 62, 71, 76, 89, 109, 120, 129, 143, 151, 191

Yogurt 5, 38, 41, 74, 89, 92, 112, 124–7, 132, 135, 137, 144, 146, 148, 155–6, 158, 160, 186, 188, 195–7